Age in Reverse

Get More Fit, Keep Your Brain Active,
and Increase Your Energy Every Day

Look and Feel Younger Than a Year Before

Steven Schuster
steveschusterbooks@gmail.com

Table of contents

Introduction

My name is Steve Schuster, and I'm 12 years old.

Before you return my book thinking that you've been the victim of a very bad joke, let me tell you, I'm indeed 12 years old—if I take my birth date strictly. I was born on February 29, 1968. Last year was the 12th occasion upon which I could really celebrate my birthday, even though I hit 50 recently.

I have to state that I neither feel nor look my age. Some say my secret is the lucky (or unlucky) fact that I was born on a leap year, and counting my actual birthdays kept my spirit young. Sure, after growing out of the elementary school "ha-ha, you're three years old" jokes, I started looking at my birth date as a blessing instead of a curse. I identified with a younger self in mind and body. I was curious how I could preserve my health and youthful looks over time. I knew I couldn't keep up with the age-divided-by-four look, per se, but I wanted to stay young since God had gifted me with an uncommon mental reassurance.

I started reading a lot about the Fountain of Youth in the late '80s and early '90s. I was fascinated to find out how age prevention techniques got discovered and contradicted during these years. However, there was not much information out there about aging, how to prevent it, and how one can improve their lifestyle to stay not only young-looking, but also mentally and physically healthy.

I come from an immigrant family. As children of immigrants may know well, our parents put in a lot of work and effort—often not considering their own health and well-being—to offer us, their children, a chance to live the American Dream.

My father was German, an accountant with a very strong work ethic. He never played with my two brothers and me. He went to work early in the morning and came home late in the evening. He was an impatient and overly exhausted man. My mother was French—a *belle* from Nice. I could write another book about the beautiful love story of my parents, which withstood the horrifying ordeals of the Second World War. A German and a

French—what irony. What an iconic cliché of the impossible relationship of those times. Their only hope for a life together was to escape to the U.S. in search of a better life.

My father came from a prosperous but simple family. His ancestors were accountants, clerks, and bankers as far back as we could track our family tree. My mother's family tree counted some nobility among them. Her family was very proud to be French. They found even the idea of a having a German commoner in the family *scandaleux*, even more so because of the postwar traumas that affected my mother's family greatly.

Being restricted by both their families and their countries, they immigrated to the United States in their late teens/early twenties. Even though they both worked very hard, they had a different approach to life. My father was not considering his health at all. He ate meat with meat, hardly slept, and was very tense all the time. Every evening when he arrived home and found no meat at the table, he used to slam it, demanding meat, saying, "*Ich bin Herr im Haus*," which in German means "I'm the master in the house." Therefore, meat was his privilege to have.

My mother, on the other hand, was very health- and beauty-conscious. She constantly tried to trick my father away from meat, fat, and sugar—but all her struggles were in vain. She was teaching French and history at one of our local schools. On the weekends, she was working as a seamstress. She was called Mrs. Pompadour at her workplaces for her stylishness, healthy looks, and always-too-busy-to-check-the-mirror behavior. She was a French lady, after all. She wore hard work with grace and class. I don't know much about what triggers mutual respect in women, but I think she was highly respected and eagerly followed by other women in the community.

I remember one day, on a sunny Friday afternoon in 1980, my father came home quite cheerful from work. This was very uncommon, considering his usual distant nature. He brought my brothers and me some ice cream from the store and sat with us in the garden, telling stories about his youth in Germany. We hung on every word he said. We were still youngsters, looking up on our father as if he was Superman himself. He was laughing and joking around in one moment, and in the next moment, he swiftly jumped up, grabbing his shirt on his left side. Then he collapsed on the ground like Goliath being struck by David.

My older brother knew what he had to do. He quickly commanded me to call my mother and for my other brother to call an ambulance while he was desperately trying to keep my father alive. It all happened so fast—the ambulance coming with its sinister siren and my mother running, screaming, and crying down the aisle of the hospital. There was nothing ladylike in her, in those moments. She looked like a mad person, grabbing the doctor's sleeves, crying, begging him to tell her good news. The doctor just shook his head, saying there was nothing to be done. My father was as good as gone. And indeed, before sunset, he was dead. Just like that. He was 45 years old.

He was strong as a bull, tall as a sequoia tree. He could lift the three of us at the same time. He always looked so healthy, even though he was tired and irritable all the time. Our family was devastated—especially my mother. She looked like a ghost. Nothing like that elegant, sassy French girl who she had been just that morning.

13

After my father died of his sudden heart attack, my mother was even more cautious to provide us with quality food, make us rest properly, and move enough. All of us started working to try to keep the family afloat. My mother started doing double shifts as a seamstress, my older brother volunteered at the local hospital, and my other brother was accepted at my father's company to work as an assistant part-time. And me, being only 12 years old, I started working as an altar boy. But I quickly realized that there are much more funerals than weddings, so I started working at funerals. Before I knew it, at the age of 12, I was spreading incense above a corpse.

My mother died last year at the age of 81 in a very unfortunate car accident, coming back from a marathon she ran at in Colorado. I'm still recovering from her loss. Objectively speaking, she was mentally and physically healthy, and if she had got the time, she would have lived 20 years more, at least.

Aging and, more specifically, how to preserve our health and young mobility occupied a significant place in my life since the moment I was born. I saw the consequence of the ignorance of self-care in my father's case when I was only 12. I also saw the opposite in my mother's case, who was still running marathons at her age.

Besides the first-hand experience I got from my parents' lifestyles, I work as a health coach. Being a former teacher, coaching doesn't stand too far from what I'm good at. I've also read more books and participated in more conferences and courses to understand human body chemistry and movement need at its core than I can count in order to have a deep knowledge about how to crack the code of aging—more specifically, how to live longer and as healthily as genetics allows, enjoying life quality on its peak, even at the age of 50 or 80.

This book will lead you through my personal experience and the experience of professional aging experts, star physicians, and other recognized names in the industry. The greatest mission of my life has been to promote healthy living. I want to help people become aware of the code of aging before it is too late. I want to do all I can to prevent another child losing his father under the tragic circumstances I did. I want to help every man and woman live with their loved ones over a long and happy life.

Born to Survive

What do you expect to change after you read this book?

Do you wish to know how to avoid some illness or reduced life quality?

Do you wish to keep your mobility longer? Do you wish to regain your mobility?

Do you fear dying? Do you have no motivation, or decreased will to be active, and you want to change that? Do you look older, feel less attractive, so you seek the Fountain of Youth?

Some people aim for healthy living in order to have a beautiful body. When I started researching and studying about aging, my primary objective was to preserve my health for as long as possible. Even before aging as a topic—or as a threatening condition—appeared in my life, I was following a healthy lifestyle, not necessarily to avoid aging, but as a consequence, I aged much slower. Just one year every four. Not quite, but almost.

The human body and brain were designed to help us survive.

If you give credit to the genetic bottleneck theory after the Toba eruption as I do, you'll realize that only a scarce amount of the human race survived it. I wondered why for a long time.

The Toba eruption was one of the biggest volcanic eruptions to date, taking place about 75,000 years ago in Indonesia, where currently, Toba Lake is situated.[i] This eruption was followed by a few years of volcanic winter and a thousand-year-long global cool down. The genetic bottleneck theory is linked to this event. The theory suggests that today's human race is a descendant of the 1000–10,000 survivors of post-Toba period.[ii]

Several archeological findings support, and some contradict, the genetic bottleneck theory. Whoever is right, one thing is true: to survive an eruption and the following drastic environmental changes as species, the body has to be extremely hardy, robust, and the brain has to be poised. Our ancestors had to adapt to the thousand-year-long climate variations.

Archeologists postulate that human species survived along the African seaside after Toba. Fish saved us. During the cool-down period, vegetables were very hard to come by. Other sources of animals were scarce, as well. Another theory suggests that we might have survived on corms. This is a starchy plant comprised mainly of carbohydrates. There is a long road here to examine why seafood became so essential for the brain.

We have smarter brains than any other species, but at the same time, our brains are fat and slow. Our brain wouldn't be able to function without the body we have. The brain-muscle signaling dominates most of our thinking. Sitting on a couch and watching TV will lead to losing your brain and skeletal muscle. The brain will start to lose its signals and degenerate. A small signal from the muscle can make the brain improve itself and maintain neurons. If muscles are disused, or underused, they begin to atrophy, or muscle cells stop repairing or replacing themselves. Both these things lead to the phenomenon we call aging.

Aging therefore is not a program, but rather the result of the failure of a renewal or repairing program. Aging is still a puzzle for neuroscientists, biochemists, and other specialists. However, it is a lot simpler than people think it to be.

Aging is not programmed. It doesn't happen by default. We don't have aging genes yet discovered. Aging is a loss of self-function, a loss of the ability of cells to renew tissues. Aging is simply damage.

The Toba eruption and the genetic bottleneck theory were meant to prove that human body and brain are highly adaptive, designed to survive, heal themselves, and be flexible to changes. We were not born to die, but to survive.

In the following chapters, I will present the biological background of aging, including the reasons for muscle atrophy, the stages of cellular function change, and how we can deter as long as possible the last stage of cell function, which is cell death.

I will talk about the best diets and exercises that can help you to put on hold your biological clock—or turn it back.

Without further ado, please let me help you.

Chapter 1: Physical Aging

Myth Buster

Hundreds of years ago, medics believed that cutting an open wound on one's arm or leg could cure certain illnesses. They also believed that homosexuality was a mental illness and that a lobotomy cures anxiety without any consequence. They were all wrong.

There are some medical theories and practices that get refuted over time. Some of the most common aging "myths" were also proven to be wrong over the course of the past few decades. My parents still believed in most of these theories when I was young. However, accelerated knowledge development in technology—including medical technology—has helped to prove these myths to be false. Let's see some of the main aging-related myths.

Myth number one: If you didn't exercise in your youth, it's too late to start in your 50s or upward.

Fact: Several experiments and studies proved this myth to be wrong. (Later in the book, I present in detail the biological background of this myth.) One particular study worked with 50 women and men with an average age of 87. Their sole task was to work out with weights for a length of 10 weeks. After the first week, the participants showed an improvement. They had more energy, could increase the repetition counts, and work with heavier weights. By the end of the 10-week trial period, the participants' muscle strength increased by 113%. They were more energized than ever, walked faster, and got tired much later than before.

Myth number two: Human brains grow only until their mid-20s. Then they slowly start to degenerate.

Fact: Neuroscientists think otherwise. They have proved that exercising is boosting the brain's plasticity.[iii] As little as 30 minutes of exercise a day can keep your brain in shape. Don't think about physical exercise only, but also mental. Do crosswords, play chess, or simply start multiplying two in your head as many times as you can.

Myth number three: Unless we won the genetic lottery, our skin will inevitably start to become the perfect imitation of a Shar-Pei as we age. We'll get wrinkles and other skin problems.

Fact: This myth is true to the point that if (unless you indeed have good genes) you don't do anything to prevent the Shar-Pei syndrome, it will get you. Thanks to today's science, however, you can delay and minimize skin-related problems if you want. You can avoid the power of gravity two ways. One, become an astronaut. Two, you can minimize gravity's impact on your skin by drinking at least eight glasses of water a day, get enough sleep, and get a good 30 minutes of exercise daily. You can protect your skin against the sun with sunscreen. Free radical activity can be balanced with a diet rich in fruits and vegetables that have free radical-fighting antioxidants. As you can see, the solution to have a healthy-looking skin actually may cost you less than a Shar-Pei dog, overall.

Myth number four: Metabolism slows down around age 40.

Fact: This myth can become reality, too, if you live a sedentary lifestyle 24/7. Without any exercise, your metabolism indeed will slow down around age 40. Studies over the past decades have proven that those people who consistently exercised at least three times a week could minimize or completely escape metabolic slowdown due to aging. They could retain their 20-year-old metabolism much longer.[iv]

Myth number five: Old people get depressed as a rule.

Fact: Adults in their twilight age, most of the time, are not depressed. When they are, it is not age-related. Depression is an illness that needs treatment, not a byproduct of aging.[v]

Next year, I will hit the age of the graceful half-century. However, I don't feel old and I don't look old. I have a few wrinkles, but not more than the average 30-year-old. And I'm more certainly not depressed. If you read this book at the age of 30 or 40, you are very lucky. You're at the right age to start taking preventive measures to minimize the effect of aging on you.

If you are 70, don't worry—you will find helpful and useful information here too. I can't promise you that my book will teleport you into your 20-year-old body, but I guarantee that you can scrub some decades off with dedication and commitment.

I'm a strong believer that how we look is less important than how we feel in our bodies. Satisfaction felt by experiencing life without the burdens of age (pain, illness, forgetfulness, and other factors) will inevitably reflect on your looks, too. My father looked like a film star, yet died in a heart attack at the age of 45. My primary goal in this book is to help you feel younger.

The good news is that if you do all you can to feel younger, those actions will make you look younger as a byproduct. If the only weapon you used against aging was a 14-karat face cream, I have bad news. It won't be enough. It might help you look younger, but it won't help your general well-being.

The Wellspring of Youth

For a long period of time, age was considered to be an inevitable, natural part of life. A few hundred years ago, people were not giving much thought about aging because very few of them lived more than 40–50 years. Thanks to the development of medicine, people's life expectancy grew exponentially. However, their quality of life expectancy didn't. Modern medicine of the past decades not only focuses on life expectancy extension, but also quality of life improvement. Today, we are very lucky to be able to access medication that helps us live longer, and tools that grant us a better quality of life, even after our glorious 30s are behind us.

Ironically, the key to our life quality increase, the eerie Fountain of Youth, was in our hands all along. Not only in our hands, but also our legs, arms, core, abs, back—everywhere we have muscles. A small part of our cells, called mitochondria, is the key to youth. Keeping your muscles young will keep you young.

The human body has an internal auto-repair program. It can relentlessly repair itself after damage. When you cut yourself, the bleeding will stop shortly, the wound will cicatrize, and depending on the size of the injury, it will slowly heal. The body can treat burn marks, agglutinate broken bones, or fight off different viruses and bacteria with its immune system. The body's main purpose is to keep you safe and, if you face any injury, to heal you as quickly as possible. Any type of physical movement aids your cellular regeneration and your adaptive responses to environmental changes.

You might think that the more well rested the body is, the more energy it has. You are correct, if by well rested you mean having had seven to eight hours of sleep. However, if during waking hours the body doesn't get active enough, it will become sluggish. The more energy you burn, the more energy you'll have in every physiological aspect.

Having strong, healthy musculature will grant you so much:

- Less pain
- Lower blood sugar
- Better circulation

- More oxygen in your body
- More energy
- Better focus
- Better memory
- Reduced risk of dementia, Alzheimer's, diabetes, high blood pressure, even cancer
- Maintenance of brain cell growth[vi]

I could go on about the benefits of physical activity and muscle maintenance. Don't feel discouraged if you are 63 and you've never had a particularly sporty life. As I said before, your body is programmed to heal and improve. You may not reach the flexibility and strength of a 63-year-old who practiced sports all his life, but you can bring out much more of your physical and cognitive abilities than you are right now. You can age 10 or even 20 years backward sooner than you'd think. Just like the folks presented in the study above, give yourself 10 weeks of a 30-minute workout at least three times a week and see the results for yourself. I strongly recommend hiring a physician or a private trainer in a gym to avoid injuries.

One of my clients is in her early 80s. She's an amazing, inspiring woman—just wonderful. She comes to my sessions two times a week and has now hired a youngster trainer, as well, who is in his mid-20s and apparently has very courteous manners. My client is reborn—not only does she feel much more energized, thanks to the weight training they do, but she also feels like a young girl when this private trainer tells her encouraging words. "That cheeky goose puts a smile on my face every Wednesday. For an hour, even though I'm 82, I feel like I'm in my 40s and act like in my 20s. What a peculiar old woman I am …" she told me once. She is peculiar in the best sense of the word.

If you are still a "cheeky goose" in your 20s or 30s, it is the right time to step on the road of agelessness. I know that at your age, it is very difficult to imagine becoming old and helpless. Billions of lives can prove, however, that this time will come unless you do something about it now. Remember about those muscles, "if you use 'em, you don't lose 'em."

Scientists suggest that only 20–30% of longevity is determined by genetics. Lifestyle choices and environmental effects determine the remaining percentage.[vii] With a little awareness and control over our diet and physical exercises, you can improve your quality of life significantly.

Aging is a natural phenomenon, indeed, but not inevitable. In her book *Aging Backwards*, Miranda Esmond-White illustrates the natural aging process through the example of a gardener. "If she tends to her garden, diligently watering her plants and ensuring they get the right amounts of sun, nutrients, and water, her plants will flourish and grow. If, however, she neglects her garden, it will soon become overgrown with weeds and, without nutrition or water, the plants will die. Both of these outcomes are equally "natural.""[viii]

Chapter 2: The Biology of Aging

How Do Cells Work?

I've always considered understanding the key to success. Before you dig yourself into something, you must have a clear knowledge of and understand the challenge you're facing; otherwise, you might fail. Just like you don't go investing on the stock market without having an idea of how the stock market works, you won't be able to fight properly against aging, either, if you don't know why you have to do certain exercises or eat some specific foods.

I know that my book might be the 10th one you read about aging, and now you might think, "Oh, I already know this." Well, on one hand, repetition is the mother of knowledge; you'll get a deeper understanding and memory about something the more you read about it. On the other hand, if you know all about aging but you're reading my book, it means you're still looking for something. Keep your mind open, and maybe you'll find it.

To learn aging fundamentals, we need to begin with a bottom-up approach. The first body parts we need to talk about are the smallest building blocks of your body—your cells.

Cells are responsible for every biological function of the human body.

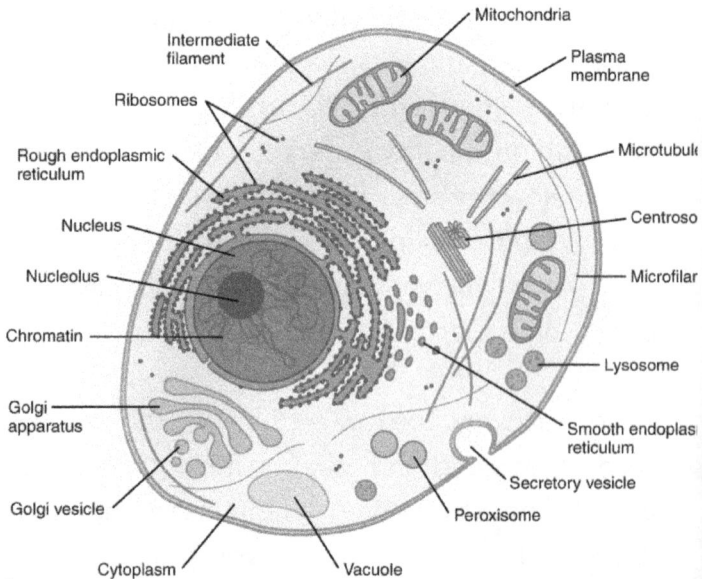

ix - *Picture I*. The Cell

As you can see in Picture 1, a cell is surrounded by plasma membrane. This plasma membrane (or cell membrane) is composed of protein and fat. Its primary function is to protect the elements inside the cell. Only a few things are allowed to enter the cell or leave the cell. Mostly food enters, and waste leaves. The inside part of the cell is filled with cytoplasm, which is a jelly-like fluid.

The nucleus, which on the picture is the big, eye-like part, is housing the DNA, our genetic code. The other function of the nucleus is to control the cell's food intake, movement, and reproduction.

If the nucleus is the mastermind of a cell, the mitochondria are the power plants. (On the picture, the mitochondria are those three striped beans from 12 to three o'clock.) To make an illustrative analogy, the mitochondria for the cell are like the heart for the body. Each cell has its own power source that energizes them and keeps them alive. There are many types of cells in the human body—stem cells, blood cells, skin cells, and so on. Most cell types have only a small number of mitochondria inside them. There is, however, one cell type that has a tremendous number of mitochondria inside. These cells hold almost 95% of human mitochondria. These are the muscle cells.[x]

Mitochondria give us energy. They are responsible for taking in nutrients. Then they use oxygen and different enzymes to break these nutrients down, creating energy for every body part. This process is called cellular respiration. The conversion of nutrients creates an energy-transfer molecule, called adenosine-triphosphate (ATP). This is a catabolic reaction, breaking large molecules into smaller ones, releasing energy in the process.

This process of generating energy, called "cellular respiration," creates ATP, an energy-transfer molecule. When a cell needs energy, the mitochondria convert carbohydrates (in the form of glycogen) or fat into energy, and then ATP shuttles the energy to whatever part of the cell needs it.[xi]

When we do something, we use some energy from our ATP stock, and to refill it, we get aided by the mitochondria. Every breath we take, every move we make, is a signal to our mitochondria, "Hey, wake up, energy is needed here." Of course, the opposite is also true. If we live a sedentary lifestyle, we message our mitochondria that we don't need their activity.

Due to physical activity, the number of mitochondria will increase in our body, and as a result, our energy will increase, as well. This explains why fit people seem to have so much energy. This explains why do you feel rejuvenated after a good, exhausting workout.

When you sit or lay most of the time, your muscles become powerless and the mitochondria's energy production stops. That's why less-fit people find they have less and less energy (what they call motivation) as days pass to get up from the couch and do something. This is why you feel overly exhausted after sitting all day. You may think, "Why am I tired? I didn't do anything all day." Well, that's precisely the reason, believe it or not.

Burn Those Calories

There are two types of muscles in your body: those that you can control voluntarily and those that are out of your control. You can control skeletal muscles like those in arms, legs, or back. You can't control your cardiac muscles, your digestive tract, your blood vessels, and so on.

Even if you don't move a bit, those uncontrollable muscles will still work relentlessly and will require energy to keep up their good work. Their mitochondria have to be fueled. The more you move, the more energy your body will require from your mitochondria. The more mitochondria activity you have, the more energized you'll feel, and last but not least, the more calories will you burn.

The body remembers. So if you don't do exercises regularly, your mitochondria production will fall back, and the smallest exercise will quickly drain the energy of your few active mitochondria. This is why people who skip the gym for one or two months complain about falling behind, getting tired easier, and a decrease in performance.

Better persist and climb those stairs, walk to that grocery instead of driving, and sweep that kitchen instead of using the robot vacuum. Stay in motion, and enjoy the simple effortlessness of everyday activities.

To illustrate the effect of mitochondria inactivity on weight gain, I'll tell you a story. Let's say your body is a fireplace. One day, the fireplace decides he doesn't want to work, doesn't want to burn any wood today. So the fireplace just rests, not burning any of the surrounding wood. However, every day the fireplace gets a new cargo of wood. If he doesn't burn any wood, the woods chunks will pile up until they run out of room. These proverbial wood chunks are the extra calories that get stored as fat everywhere. How can the fireplace get rid of the extra wood? By starting to burn them. There is new wood cargo coming every day, anyway.

Now, let's change a letter in the example and turn wood into food. The art of weight loss is simple mathematics. If you consume more food (calories) than what you burn, there will be an excess energy source around that your body will store. For example, you can go for an hour run and burn 800 calories if you eat a copious pork chop with bread and mustard afterward. Then the calories you just burned with the one-hour effort will invade your body again.

If your aim is to lose weight, exercise alone is not enough. You can't run a race with a beef stew splashing in lard. You can't burn 2000–3000 calories a day. You'll have to mind your diet and daily calorie intake to stabilize, or lose weight.

There is, however, a little trick that can help you burn more calories: focus on your large muscle groups for enhanced calorie burn. Our thighs, abdominal muscles, and hips are among those muscles that we call large muscles. They have more mitochondria than smaller muscle groups; therefore, stimulating them with exercise will lead to more calories burned.[xii]

Why Does the True Battle Against Aging Start in Our 40s?

Exercise helps you to keep your cells alive by giving your mitochondria a reason to live. This is even more important after the age of 40 when, due to lack of movement, cells atrophy—or die. After the age of 40, if the mitochondria don't feel needed, it will slowly shut itself down. While the activity level of an average 40-year-old decreases, their appetite—their food intake—stays the same. Since there are fewer mitochondria to take care of the food burning, the excess will inevitably show itself all around the body. We call this phenomenon *metabolism slowdown due to aging*, but it's rather due to lack of mobility. In fact, what's happening is as simple as this: you let your cells atrophy, you have fewer mitochondria to burn your unchanged food portions, and you gain weight.

People consider the age of 40 the metabolic bugaboo. Those who have been mindful about nutrition and motion don't have to stress about meeting the bugaboo. But those who didn't take care of themselves will start to experience the capital-lettered Aging. The two biggest hits they'll suffer are atrophy and cell death.

Let's take a microscopic look at how our life starts. When we hit the proverbial start mark in the race called life, we are nothing more than the combination of two cells: a sperm and an egg. Right after the start, these cells start multiplying like crazy, generating more and more cells that form our body parts. Trillions of different cells (muscle, brain, blood, nerve, and other cells) multiply to make each stage of our life happen. We grow visibly month by month as a child, and we start to be more feminine or masculine as years go by.

Cells, however, don't live forever. They die, and new cells are created. It is a constant cycle. Up to the age of 14, people lose 30–40 billion cells a day, but new ones are equally generated. When we are "ready," in a cell-sense (around the age of 20), we jump into a new phase of cellular activity—the repairing and replacement process. Apoptosis, the process of programmed cell death, speeds up to 50–70 billion death cells a day. This acceleration serves to maintain homeostasis.

The process of repairing and replacement goes on steadily until the mesmeric age of 40. However, at that age, we hit another life stage milestone. By the time we reach this milestone, our cells have divided so many times that they become a bit gawky. Why is that?

Because each time the cells divide, they nip off the protective caps at the end of the chromosome while they copy the DNA. By the time we are 40, our cells have divided 40–50 times, and the chromosome protecting caps (telomeres) almost disappeared. Therefore, the body gets the message to stop cell division. At this point, we enter the "cellular senescence" stage, which in practice is the death of cells.[xiii]

42

Experts today believe more and more that mitochondrial function holds the solution to slowing down aging. If we can prevent mitochondria from decreasing in number and preserve their health, it can significantly improve our quality of life and keep us healthy for much longer.

As I said before, what we inherited in our DNA determines about 30% of our fate. The rest of our fate is the result of how we take care of our body and depends singularly on the choices we make. When I'm talking about choices, sometimes they mean as little as taking the stairs, not the elevator, choosing to stand instead of sitting, eating more fruits, avoiding direct exposure to the sun, stressing less, and sleeping an extra hour. All these small actions take a lot of the burden off our genetic shoulders.

Besides these small steps of protection, we can take clear action to protect our cellular health and prevent premature aging. You might not like this part, but if you want to stay young for long, you can't skip it. It's exercising. Regular exercise increases in our body an enzyme called telomerase. Telomerase is responsible for protecting our telomeres by improving mitochondrial function and preventing mitochondrial loss and cell death. Therefore, if we exercise, telomerase will keep our mitochondrial functions alive for longer, deterring aging as a result.

As we hit the age of 40, if the body is not used to exercise, the message not to replace or repair cells will spread and strengthen. This means that the process of cellular senescence gets more intense and accelerated each year after 40. Each physiological aspect of the body starts to decline as a consequence, as well. Our heart becomes weaker, and our lungs won't function as well as they did before, either. Female estrogen and male testosterone levels will decrease, just to mention a few aspects of aging—which are well known to many of us.

Although scientists still don't have a crystal-clear answer on how to stop the process we call aging, there are some questions answered on the matter. For example, how do you keep your cells in the repairing and replacing phase for longer, instead of letting them die? The answer is quite simple—you have to prove to your body that you still need your cells to repair and replace themselves, and that you need energy. How can you prove it? By exercising. And not only exercising, but also moving each muscle that you want to preserve from aging. For example, if you walk only, muscle cells in your legs might stay active, but this won't prevent other muscle cells from atrophying in other parts of your body. You need to move all the 620 skeletal muscles in your body.

Beware Atrophy

Cell death is not the only way your body can lose cells. Keeping cellular repairing and replacing is not the only problem you should address with exercise—especially after a certain age.

The other issue is atrophy.

Atrophy is the wasting away of the body or of an organ or limb. Atrophy can occur due to bad nutrition, nerve damage, lack of exercise, or other reasons. Healthy cells shrink until they completely disappear. If the cells disappear, that means the mitochondria within will disappear, as well. The fewer mitochondria we have, the less energy we'll have. The less energy we have, the less we'll move. The less we move ... you know what happens: loss of teeth, hair, weight, bad brain functions, wrinkles, and weakness will destroy our everyday lives at old age.

A sedentary lifestyle is the most common reason for muscular atrophy. Couch potatoes, clerks, and all those people who spend most of their day in horizontal or sitting positions are at the greatest risk of developing muscular atrophy. Since they sit so much, they won't have energy. If they don't have energy, they won't feel the call to move. They'll get through the day sitting chair to chair.

Atrophy is a slow process. You won't feel a harsh dong in your head when it starts to happen. When you become aware of it, sometimes it is too late to do anything about it. This is why I want to raise your awareness about atrophy. If you are over 30 and you spend most of your day sitting, it's time to take measures against it, because you're in great danger of developing muscular atrophy. Muscle atrophy occurs when you don't use the muscle enough. If you've noticed you hunch your back often, your movements are stiffer than before, you have trouble getting out of the bed or a car, your walking pace is slowed down, or you have restricted range of motion, there is a chance that you are in the beginning stage of muscular atrophy.

There is another cause for muscle atrophy called neurogenic atrophy. It occurs more suddenly than atrophy due to muscle underuse. This type of atrophy can develop as the result of an injury or a disease of a nerve that connects to the muscle, and it is the most severe type of muscle atrophy.[xiv] For example, when you break your arm or leg, the healing process can take weeks, and the rehabilitation process can take months. After your limb gets out of the cast, it appears much slimmer than your other, healthy limb. That is the result of neurogenic muscle atrophy.

In this book, I focus on muscle atrophy rooted in muscle disuse—simple human negligence.

Muscle atrophy can be divided into three stages. In the first stage, motion seems more difficult and exhausting than before. In stage two, people can't move their muscles individually, but with the help of somebody else, they can still make the simplest motions. In stage three, muscles are immovable.

At this stage, the damage is irreversible—the muscles are totally atrophied.

The third stage can't be helped, but the other two stages can be reversed with dedication to motion. It doesn't even have to be a great effort, just baby steps—literally. Walk first, then jog, and then run. The more you move, the more the shrunken cells will become energized. Atrophy will be reversed, and you'll get supplied with more and more energy.

In your daily exercise routine, try to mobilize as many muscles as possible. If you walk only, your upper body muscles won't be trained thoroughly. If you do sit-ups or a different kind of core exercise, other muscle groups will be unattended.

With Arnold Schwarzenegger, bodybuilding became a ... thing. While doing heavy weight lifting can turn your body into a statue worthy of an Italian sculptor, it has its disadvantages. Exercising with weight on targeted muscle groups is a concentric type of training. It means that muscles get shortened or contracted. After years of concentric exercising, the muscle will prevent you from having a full range of motion, will squeeze the joints, and will cause pain. If you are a devoted member of the gym, be aware that having overbuilt musculature can also lead to atrophy. Due to overtraining, the muscles become immobile and inflexible.

The Human Oil

Not every kind of motion is good for us long-term, but it is still better to move than not to move at all. Autopsies revealed that those people who lived a sedentary lifestyle had much more hardened fat around their organs and throughout their body than those who were active.

Our fascia has a natural lubrication system, an oil that connects the musculoskeletal system. This oil is produced relentlessly, 24/7, in our bodies, nourishing our musculature, cells, and bones and helping us to move smoothly. This oil prevents our cells from adhering to each other, lubricating their external cell membranes. If this didn't happen, the cells would stick together, making us stiff, which is a common characteristic of advanced age.

This oil, however, has a very oil-like characteristic. Just like coconut oil or lard, if it is not used, it solidifies. Without regular motion, our fascia oil doesn't get softened and absorbed by the body. Instead, it will stiffly cover the muscles, making them lazy and sluggish. This hardened oil tells long tales for pathologists. The best way to keep our body well-oiled is to move consistently.

I know, by the way, that you'd like to read about a different solution that doesn't involve motion at all. Many of my clients complain to me how miserable they feel just at the notion that they have to do some motion all their lives. They try to trick me into a more appealing answer with tricky questions. When I say that the solution to their problems are specific exercises (that I will present in detail later in this book), they ask me, sheepishly, frequently nodding and wringing their hands, "I'm sure there must be another solution. Right? *Right*?"

Sure, there are other practices they can do to improve their life quality even more, but no solution package will exclude exercising. It is simple biology. That's why I thought to present these biological reasons thoroughly, so you believe me when I say that exercising is really the Fountain of Youth. If you already have felt pain, you must certainly know that there are struggles way worse than a 30-minute physical activity.

Body oils lubricate our cells each minute of the day, and this means they lubricate them even while we sleep. For seven or eight long hours, we don't move at all to smoothen these oils. This explains why we feel so stiff in the mornings, and why morning workouts are so efficient. If we stimulate the mildly stiffened oil to absorb into our cells, we'll feel much more mobile, flexible, and energized.

If you are out of shape, you probably don't feel too much mental or physical desire to move more. This attitude must be broken voluntarily; otherwise, your body oil will keep stiffening and you'll be even less energized and rigid. The more this process evolves, the less mental power you will have to break out of this vicious circle. One day, you'll open your eyes and say, "Man, I'm old."

It shouldn't be this way. You shouldn't feel this way. This condition is not genetics, and it is not fate—it is simple, self-induced atrophy.

Movement is essential to avoid illnesses and aging. It is also essential for healing.

As I said, not only sedentary lifestyles can lead you to the slippery slope of aging. So can certain exercises (like overdone concentric trainings) or proper trainings with bad equipment, things you usually pay a lot of money for because you think it is the best you can give to your body—stuff like orthopedic shoes or high-end running shoes with ankle protection padding. It sounds counterintuitive, I know, but let's take a closer look on what happens with your leg in these shoes. Your joints and muscles get accustomed to the padding of these shoes, and before you know it, they become dependent on the support these shoes offer. Some muscles won't have to work anymore; therefore, they get weaker and start to atrophy.

If you just bought some magic shoe for a four-figure price, don't get too sad about it. They are certainly helpful, to an extent. All you have to do is to balance their effect. How? By walking barefoot for half an hour at home. This inexpensive exercise can compensate for the tension-releasing effect of the different orthopedic shoes. Also, if you like to run—regardless if it is a hobby or you do it on a professional level, avoid hard surfaces. Always go to a special running track developed for this purpose, or run in nature on real earthy ground. Hard and stiff material like concrete will cause you joint trauma. Being overweight can also damage your joints and make you feel stiff, inflexible, in pain, and, ultimately, old.

Stretching exercises pull the joints apart, preventing joint damage. If joints are pulled apart, there is more space for the aforementioned body oil to lubricate. In the following chapters, I will talk about the best stretching exercises that can help you stay fit, flexible, and young.

Chapter 3: "Flexability"

Unchain Your Muscles

Flexibility—or as I call it, "flexability"—the ability to be flexible—is key to living a full and happy life. There's a saying among physicians, namely that "you are only as loose as your tightest muscle." Regardless of how flexible your body is, if any small muscle of a joint is too tight or weak to hold the joint correctly, the tightest muscle will pull the joint out of line, unbalancing it and causing pain. This little tight muscle can make your day miserable. Therefore, I find it essential to have each skeletal muscle stretched and strengthened. Balancing your muscular structure is a life-changing magic.

Lower body blockages, like stiffness in ankles, affect how we walk and how much energy we have available. Stiffness in the ankles causes tension in the calf muscles. Any weakness or lack of flexibility can spread into seemingly unrelated parts of the body, causing pain. Upper body blockages will result in problems like back pain, tight legs, poor posture, drooping shoulders, or a hunched back that leads to pain. Your least flexible muscle will dictate your range of motion.

The Power of the Muscles

Muscles are our auto-installed superpower. They help us change locations, supply our body with energy, keep us in shape, and give us shape, for that matter. When I talk about muscles, I refer to the following: the skeletal muscles made of billions of muscle cells and hard-working mitochondria, and the tendons that attach the muscles to the bones.

The only thing we can change about our overall physical appearance is the shape of our muscles. We can't really help our height or our bone structure, can we? Each muscle we have is equally important, serving a clear purpose in our body. Having a full-body workout with total muscle involvement not only saves the muscle cells from atrophy, but also reduces stress and improves mitochondrial functions. By now, we have concluded that these are big triggers for aging.

What is considered a full-body workout with full muscle involvement? Remember how you used to play when you were a kid? You probably were limbs all around, running, jumping, crawling, and doing a large variety of other movements. As a kid, you knew how to do a proper full-body workout better than you probably do now.

Adults of the previous centuries had their own sets of full-body motions in forms of chores. That's right, those horrible chores were good for something, namely to keep your body in shape. When people swept, lots of muscles contributed to this motion. Arms, legs, and torso were working together to clean the kitchen. Making the bed needed your arms, abs, and back to collaborate. However, machines slowly took over everyday chores. On one hand, this made our lives much easier and saved a lot of our time. But on the other hand, it fostered us—especially Westerners—from our daily must-be-done-or-what-will-the-neighbors-say motions.

Chores were great to do isotonic movements. Isotonic means "equally resistant." For example, when we washed clothes, we used our shoulders, abs, and back muscles. Tension in the muscle remained constant while it shortened and lengthened—we had to hold the cloth, rub it, and squeeze it at the end. The steps of washing all involved isotonic contractions.

Today is more about concentric, or positive training. The best visual example I can give is when we lift weights at the gym. During concentric movement, the muscle shortens while under tension. Weight lifting, tennis, football, and hockey are all motions that use concentric muscle strengthening. Why? Because most of these sports require power generation through bent joints. You pull the muscles toward the center of your body. Concentric movements develop the Arnold-like bulky muscles.

The third method of exercise is doing eccentric movements, or negative training. In this sense, "negative" doesn't mean "bad." In fact, especially after a certain age, this type of movement is the best for the body. Here the muscles extend and lengthen due to contraction. For example, when you lower the weight you used for biceps training, the bicep muscles will lengthen while remaining contracted. This is what eccentric movement means.

Muscles contract when they move and relax when the motions are finished. Due to contraction, muscle fibers slide together, and when the motion is done, they slide apart. The important part of this story is that muscles have only a limited range of how far can they slide. People regularly use up to 40% of their muscles' sliding ability since everyday tasks (especially since we don't have to do all the chores with human power) don't need our full use of muscular flexibility or strength.

However, to have a good posture, be pain-free long-term, and age gracefully, we need a muscle sliding capacity minimum of 50–70% range of motion. And we need to have this capacity in all of our muscles. As we saw above, if muscles don't move, they atrophy and muscle cells die. And that leads to aging. To age slower and better, we need strength, flexibility, and endurance in our musculature. We need them, not only to age better, but also to be able to do our daily tasks easily.

Why? Because if we have power, it means we can lift heavy objects easily. If we have endurance, it means that we can carry the heavy object from the kitchen to the car. In other words, we can sustain effort for a longer time.

How can we get better at them? You can develop power if you repetitively do motions with weights. Endurance is cultivated by doing slow and steady activities. Running, swimming, and cycling (commonly known as cardio exercises) help you improve your endurance. But sweeping, weeding your garden, or washing your car can also add to it.

As we grow older, our power and endurance capacities decrease. While in our youth, it was easy to increase them both, but when we grow older, we have to put effort into maintaining or improving them. Approaching the subject from the other angle—in order to stay physically young as you age, you have to increase both your power and endurance trainings.

If you got scared of this information, don't worry. You don't have to lift heavier each week or run a marathon distance daily. Increase your power and endurance trainings over time, at least in the beginning. You can also "improve" your training by walking a little bit faster. This simple change will improve not only your endurance, but also the power of your lower body. Walking downhill is a very good eccentric exercise, and much less tiring than walking uphill.

Make your everyday motions bigger. When you cook, imagine you're the hero or heroine of a Shakespearean drama. Take the pepper from the shelf with an exaggerated range of motion. Put it back, then take it off again. Make bigger, rather than smaller, moves.

The older we get, the more we have to face and fight conditions like nutrient deficiencies, infections, falls, or other traumatic injuries, decreasing cardiac capacities, and other problems. In the United States, one of the most common reasons why older people get hospitalized is congestive heart failure. This means the heart can no longer pump enough blood throughout the body. The condition results in weakness, fatigue, low sodium and hemoglobin levels, and, ultimately, coma or death.

What's the best way to maintain your cardiovascular system? Exercising. A good 20- to 30-minute exercise a day can do the trick. Walking, stretching, or weight workouts are equally good. Strength training is one of the best ways to keep your heart strong and pumping. Unarguably, the heart is our most important muscle, and our musculature plays an important role in keeping the cardiovascular system functioning normally. How? Muscles in motion are designed to act as pumps and help the blood circulate in our veins. This pumping action of the muscles helps the blood vessels to deliver blood, unloading them partially of their pumping duty.

The vessels can't do as good of a job without the muscles helping them. If the vessels are "left alone" to deliver the blood, some cells might not receive enough nutrients or fresh blood rich in oxygen. Those cells can be exposed to chronic tiredness (somewhat like when you can't get enough sleep for weeks in a row).

The circulatory system has two tasks: (1) to deliver oxygen-rich blood to each cell in the body and (2) to wash out all the toxins, dead cells, and wastes. If the circulatory system is lazy, biologically it means it doesn't deliver enough oxygenated blood and doesn't clean out enough toxins. As a result, we'll feel tired, our skin will look lifeless, and so on.

Continuous research in the field of circulatory health showed that a type of protein called myokines[xv] is released due exercise. This protein goes from the muscle through the bloodstream and sets off changes in cells other than the ones in which they were released.

Having good circulation is the best blush and face cream, I'd say. And good circulation can be granted with as little as 10 minutes of large body movements every day. This way you increase blood flow, clear out your toxins, and fill your body with oxygen. A study at Harvard Medical School proved that tai chi and movements alike are very effective in preventing coronary artery defects. They can also improve cholesterol levels and regulate blood pressure at a lower level.

Keep Your Balance

Falling over and suffering a more severe injury is very dangerous, especially for the elderly. If an old person breaks their leg, it will take them considerably more time to recover than it would a young person. Muscle atrophy will be much harder to reverse, because at that point, cells shrink and die rather than repair or replace themselves. A serious fall, like one that results in a hip injury, sometimes can lead to total muscle degeneration, which leads to mental degeneration and death.

To prevent this, elderly people have to start recovering and moving as soon as possible after any injury—go to rehabilitation, and a physician if needed. An even better prevention is a de facto prevention—increasing your fast-twitch muscle fiber. These fibers are mostly known for their importance in jumping, running, or heavy weight lifting, but it is also critical to have them to "catch us" before we fall over.

Balance Your Mind

Recent studies have proven that exercising helps not only your body, but also your mind. In other words, exercising protects your neurological system and is a good antidepressant and focus-booster. Exercise keeps the brain in shape—literally. It commands our stem cells to create new neurons. And as you may know by now, the more cells we have, the more mitochondria we'll have. The more mitochondria, the more energy the brain will have.

A big risk of aging is falling over. As mentioned earlier in this chapter, a serious fall can be fatal to the elderly. Therefore, it is essential to keep our balance as we age. Even if we don't fall over, without a good balance, everyday actions will prove to be real challenges. Riding a bus, playing with grandchildren, or simply getting out of the bed can become serious nightmares. Without good balance, we become vulnerable, dependent on the help of others, and anxious about our safety.

What's the solution? Exercise. More precisely, balance-improving exercises. We tend to overestimate how much balancing exercise we do in our adulthood. As a child, I used to walk on train lines, very narrow trees, jump around, and fearlessly climb onto everything that invited my sense of adventure. As I grew older, obviously I didn't monkey around on the railroads anymore; I skipped the climbing, jumping, and narrow path-walking, as well. I did nothing to challenge my balance. Therefore, the balance connections in my brain started to erode. After all, as a responsible adult, I should have been seeking safety instead of instability—or so I thought.

The problem with the nerve fibers responsible for balance reflexes is that after a certain age, they can't improve. From that point on, we have to make our best effort to keep whatever balance reflexes we've developed up to that point. The nerve cells we lose are gone forever. Maintaining balance reflexes is not a joke; you'd better start working on them today, because tomorrow, you'll have less to save.

How to Improve Your Balance

You can start with very simple exercises, like standing on one leg close to the wall where you can support yourself, if necessary. Safety prevails. Go next to the wall, or a strong table (don't do this exercise with a chair; it is unsafe), hold it with your left hand, and slowly lift your right leg behind you. When you feel balanced, release the wall or table and try to stay on one leg for as long as you can (no longer than one minute). Support yourself, if necessary. Then repeat the exercise, switching your hand and leg. Do a total of three repetitions on each leg.

When you feel more comfortable and in balance, try to put your leg on the knee of your other leg, forming the shape of number four with them. Hold this position from 30 seconds to one minute. Stay close to a table or the wall to be able to support yourself, if necessary. If you feel a sharp pain in your legs or back, stop the exercise immediately.

Another version of this exercise is to write the letters of the alphabet with one leg inclined at a 45-degree angle. Keep a support close to avoid falling, but try to make as much progress through the alphabet as possible without support.

Balancing exercises are very simple, and it is never too late to start them. The best thing about them is that they are free; you can do them anywhere there is a wall or table, and they take five to 10 minutes of your life.

Scientists have proven that balance-improving exercise types such as yoga or tai chi actually help maintain or improve brain capacity and memory, and prevent the development of dementia.

Digestion

What Happens When We Digest?

Our digestive system breaks food into molecules that can be absorbed by our cells and burned in our mitochondria to supply us with energy. Digestion is also important for getting nutrients the body uses for growth and cell repair or replacement. The digestive system breaks down nutrients into carbohydrates, protein, fats, and vitamins.

Digestion works by moving food through the gastrointestinal (GI) tract. Digestion starts within the mouth and ends in the small intestine. The food, once chewed and swallowed, goes through the esophagus. As it arrives in the stomach, it mixes with digestive juices. Here, the large molecules of food break down into smaller molecules that get absorbed in the small intestine. These small molecules get into the bloodstream, which delivers each type of molecule to their proper place. Any waste after digestion goes to the large intestine and leaves the body in the form of stool.[xvi]

Picture II: The digestive system[xvii]

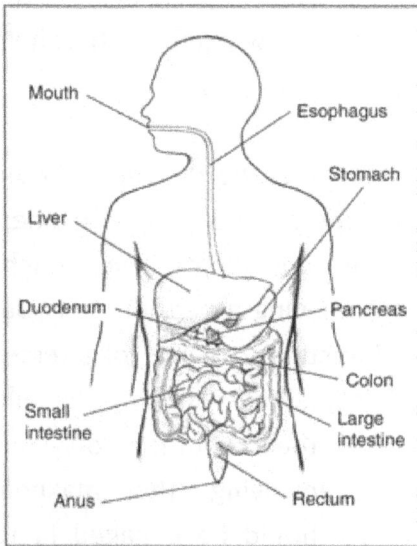
The digestive system

The digestive system is located in the torso. When we are born, we have enough space to house our digestive system inside our body and ensure its effective functioning. However, if with aging we start to develop poor posture, our digestive system might get squeezed, thus losing its efficiency. If the upper part of the digestive system gets squeezed, problems like acid reflux, heartburn, or choking might occur. If the lower part has insufficient space, you might experience constipation and poor elimination. Maintaining good posture is essential to maintaining healthy digestion with age.

How Can You Improve Your Posture?

By strengthening the muscles in your torso. In the next chapter, I'll present a few exercises that help strengthen and lengthen your torso.

To achieve smooth digestion, you should strengthen your muscles around your intestines. When you feel swollen and bloated, you might think your stomach is playing a bad joke on you. But in reality, your intestines are the jokesters—they are bloating, twisting, and twitching like wild dancers. To improve the condition of your intestines, exercises involving the maximal twisting of your torso should be engaged in to ease the loosening of intestines and help elimination. I will present a good exercise for this in the next chapter.

The need for good posture goes beyond having a good digestive system. A straight back gives you the appearance of confidence and vivaciousness. Opening up your body gives your organs place to function, while a hunched back squeezes the organs, forcing them to push outward, making you seem fatter than you are. What can your poor organs do if they have nowhere to go? They go where they can, transforming your body into the shape of an ogre.

But how poor posture makes us look is the least of our concerns. Our lungs won't be able to supply our brains with sufficient oxygen, which will lead to fatigue and slowness. Poor posture affects the work of the cardiovascular system, as well. It won't be able to provide us with proper circulation, and thus, we won't get enough energy-giving blood. I hope these are enough reasons for you to improve your posture.

The Importance of Lean Muscles

A recent discovery by the *American Journal of Clinical Nutrition* suggests that lean muscle mass is "inversely correlated with mortality in over 1000 men with an average age of 82.1." Maintaining muscle seems to be your best bet to tapping into the proverbial Fountain of Youth and aging healthily. The study didn't find the same correlation in women; however, lean muscle has anti-aging benefits for everyone.[xviii]

Eccentric exercises are perfect for the purpose of developing lean muscles. I work out almost every day, focusing on eccentric exercises for 24 minutes. When I say eccentric exercises, I mean weightlifting in negative. It is difficult to do some exercises in negative if you don't have a training partner. They can cause injuries, so don't do them alone above a certain weight. All muscle groups respond positively to negative training, so feel free to ask your personal trainer (if you have one) for tailor-made eccentric exercises. I highly recommend hiring a personal trainer to avoid injuries, especially if you are above a certain age.

In the next chapter, I will present some risk-free eccentric exercises for lean muscle-building. However, for better and faster results, I advise you to consult a physician or personal trainer. In this book, I focus on giving tips to the vast majority of people—who are relatively healthy, maybe not as fit as they could be, but are not suffering from any special condition. If you have an injury or other physical problem that calls for special exercises (or nutrition), please take this book as an information manual and always consult your doctor before applying any advice herein.

When you start practicing any kind of eccentric exercise, don't push yourself too hard—especially in the beginning. "Beginning" can mean two weeks to two months, depending on your fitness level. If you are more or less fit, after two weeks you can become 10% cockier than before. If you are absolutely out of shape, getting over the starting phase can take up to two months. Don't overdo it with the timeframe of the exercises, either. In the beginning, start gently, with a maximum 30 minutes of training. As a matter of fact, you'll strengthen your muscles quicker if you work out while relaxed and not overexerting yourself. Why? Because if you want to do too much too quickly, you may get discouraged and quit.

Walk slower, get farther. That's my motto in building lean muscles.

Attention: Whenever you feel a sharp pain in your body while doing any exercise, stop doing it immediately. There is a difference between "normal" pain you might feel, like being sore or simply inflexible, and a deep, knifelike pain. If you feel the latter and don't stop the exercise, you may end up with an injury.

Fitness to Defeat Fatness

Here are two key takeaways you should keep in mind about the relation of exercise to weight loss.

First, work out all your 620 muscles to keep your calorie-burning mitochondria alive by preventing muscles from atrophying. To speed up calorie burning, you need to turn up mitochondrial activity, and to do this, you need to move. But moving in a certain manner burns even more calories than usual. This affirmation leads us to the second takeaway.

Second, active, large muscles burn more calories. The abdominals, quadriceps, gluteus muscles, and hamstrings form your large muscles. The more you engage them in your workout, the more calories will you burn.

Prevent poor posture, prevent cell death, and prevent atrophy to stay young longer and age better. Exercising is the key to preventing these three tragedies that will surely lead you to quick and painful aging.

Check with a doctor about your current physical condition. Do not try to self-diagnose based on this book. Everything I wrote here is for the sake of information. No book can accurately draw up seven billion personal conditions. If you experience pain, chronic exhaustion, or other abnormalities, it could be because of a wealth of reasons too numerous to describe here. A doctor can give you an accurate diagnosis and plan to follow for recovery. What you read in this book is me offering suggestions on how to prevent or improve general age-related conditions. I cannot predict your accurate physical condition through paper; therefore, I don't want to give specific advice, either.

Your body is designed to be well-balanced, flexible, strong, and self-healing. If you start "repairing" the damage you've done to it over the years, your body will swiftly respond to the positive stimuli. You might not become 20 again, but with devotion to exercise for only 30 minutes a day, you'll be able to feel good again and do things you didn't dare for a long time. Make this 30-minute workout your top priority every day and enjoy the benefits you'll reap.

Chapter 4: Exercises

Before we jump into the middle of the exercises, I'd like to say a few words of caution about stretching. The warning does not apply to all exercises below, just to those that are typical stretching exercises. To properly execute stretching exercises, four things should be taken into consideration:

1. Hold the stretch long enough

Hold the stretched position for at least 10–15 seconds before you return to your starting position. Why? Because if you don't hold the stretched position long enough, you may start bouncing, which can result in injury. People tend to rush through the stretching part of a workout, which is quite the opposite of what stretching should be about.

2. Bouncing

Most people are mistakenly convinced that bouncing is the key to a good stretch. The problem with bouncing is that you do a lot of damage when you try to push your muscles beyond their natural reflex. Make consistent, smooth stretching moves. Push yourself only until you feel a mild tension, hold that position for 10–15 seconds, and then release it. The more you stretch, the more flexible you'll become—with time.

3. Overstretching

Never push yourself more than feels natural. Make your stretching workout challenging, but never overstep that proverbial—and literal—sharp pain line. Stretching is about relaxation, not high performance. Give yourself the time to do the routine smoothly and gently. Your muscles are attached to tendons. The tendons hold the muscle to the bone. Attaching the muscle to the tendon is a muscle roll, which is quite sensitive to stretch. Avoid overstretching to prevent causing injury to your tendons.

4. Losing focus on the form

Before you start stretching, think through which muscles you will be using for your workout, or which muscles you did use. Different types of workouts call for different types of stretching. For example, if you go running, you have to warm up your legs and lower body, mostly. If you do an upper body workout with weights, a different type of stretching is required. Pay attention to your muscles and focus on maintaining the correct posture. Since stretching is stationary and you have to hold a pose for several seconds, your mind might wander. Prevent this. Focus on the muscle and pay attention to what your stretching limit is—that is, the point that gives you a good kind of pain, not a bad kind. Correct your stretching posture, if needed.

We become weaker as we age. This means that our cells become weaker, as well. That's why gravity's effect starts to show on us more visibly— for example, in the form of saggy skin on our arms, which I call waving elephant ears.

With a little bit of extra effort and awareness, however, Dumbo-ear arms are preventable. There is a very good, and ridiculously easy, exercise you can do to prevent it.

First Block of Exercises: Ditching Dumbo

Collect the Apples

Lift your arms above your head. Stretch upward to lengthen the muscles of the trunk and back at the same time. Gravity pulls your vertical muscles down; therefore, you have to balance this effect by stretching upward. Training the large vertical muscles in the spine daily will slow down the effect of gravity.

First, lift both your arms above your head. Imagine that you want to reach some apples on a tall tree, so try to stretch upward to get it first with one hand, then the other. Do not force the motion. Stretch only as much as it feels natural to avoid injuries. Repeat the stretching 15 times with both arms. When you're done, release your arms. Rest for a minute, then do it again. Repeat the exercise four times in total. This exercise shouldn't take more than eight minutes—about one minute of activity and one minute of rest.

Arm Swing

When you've collected all the apples on the imaginary tree, move on to the next DD (Ditching Dumbo) exercise. Swing your right arm toward the ceiling with a wide range of motion and let it down. While you let down your right arm, lift your left arm the same way you did your right. Then switch them again. Repeat this arm swing exercise 20 times on each side for a total of 40 swings. Rest for 30 seconds and do it again. Repeat the exercise four times in total.

Arm Stretching

After you're finished with the arm swing lift, put your right arm above your head and try to reach the ceiling. But this time, don't let it down. Reach toward the ceiling as much as you can, breathing deeply. As you inhale, stretch your arm higher. As you exhale, release the tension in your muscles and stop stretching. Repeat three times.

After you're done with the inhale-exhale upward arm stretch, don't let your arm down. Pull the same arm gently backward. Do not exaggerate. This should be a very small range of motion. If you do it correctly, you should feel a smooth traction in your frontal shoulder joint. Hold this pose for five seconds while you inhale, then gently exhale, slowly dropping your arm. Repeat the same exercise with your left arm. Repeat the practice 10 times on both sides.

Arm stretching won't only help you with the gravity, but will also strengthen your back, improving your posture.

Second Block of Exercises: Torso Strengthening—Lengthening

Stretching Cat

If you do yoga, you might be familiar with this exercise. Use a yoga mat to avoid pain in your knees and palms. This exercise targets the cartilage in the backbone, flexing it every time you perform it. It is also an effective exercise to stretch your lower back muscles. Caution: if you have chronic back or knee pain, do not try this exercise, or otherwise, consult with your doctor before doing so.

To perform the exercise, get on your hands and knees. Place your hands parallel to your shoulders. Lock your arms out. While you inhale, flex your spine down and bring your head up. Exhale while you arch your spine up and bring your head down. Repeat this 10 times. Rest for a minute while you sit on your mat. Repeat this exercise four times.

Side Leg Lifts

When you're finished with the stretching cat exercise, it's time to work on those legs a bit. Lay down on your yoga mat on your left side, supporting the pose with your left arm lifted, putting your head on it, and placing your right arm in front of you. Lift both of your legs as high as you can while keeping your upper body on the floor. Do not exaggerate the motion. If you can lift your legs only a little bit, that's fine too. Gently put your legs back to the starting position. Feel as your upper and lower body lengthen away from each other. Repeat lifting your legs five to eight times, then switch sides and do the same. When you're done, rest lying on your back for a minute. Repeat the exercise four times on both sides.

Pretzel Exercise

Sit on the yoga mat, putting your left leg out in front and bending it while holding the ankle of your right leg with your right hand. Keep your right leg to the back, also bent. Pull your heel gently toward your butt. Make sure to put your body weight on the thigh, not the knee. Hold the stretching position for 10–15 seconds, then gently release the stretched leg. Repeat three times on this side, then switch sides and repeat it on the other side as well.[xix]

Dry Swimming

Dry swimming is one of the most effective upper body stretching exercises. It moves all the muscles of the upper body, including hip muscles. The exercise stretches the lower back very effectively and relieves back pain. It might cause a gentle soreness in your back for the next two days, but hey, that means you did a great job. If, however, you feel a sharp pain during or after the exercise, stop doing it and turn to your doctor.

Lie on your stomach with your legs and arms straight on the ground. Your arms should be above your head. Lie in a straight line like an arrow. Raise your left arm and right leg diagonally from your body and hold position for 10 seconds. Gently release your limbs and relax for a few seconds. Then switch to the right arm / left leg and repeat the exercise. Do a maximum of three repetitions on both sides, then stand up and relax for a minute. Repeat this exercise three times on both sides.

Stretching Cobra

Your last exercise in torso strengthening and posture improving is another yoga pose called the stretching cobra. It targets mainly the muscles in the middle of the back. It also stretches the abdominal muscles and the cartilage in the spinal cord.

This exercise might cause pain and resistance in the beginning, but as you get used to it, the resistance and pain will dissolve. I still don't mean the sharp, knife-like pain—just a gentle one. If you feel a sharp pain, stop the exercise immediately.

Lie on your stomach on the yoga mat. Put your hands under your shoulders, your fingers facing forward. Keep your legs straight and your toes pointed.

While you exhale, press your hips into the mat, lengthen your torso, and lift your chest, curling up from the ground while your hips stay stable. Support yourself on your arms. Raise your head and look upward. Stretch in this pose for as long as it remains comfortable. Hold this position for 10–15 seconds. When you're done, gently lower your upper body back to the mat. Lengthen your spine as you descend.

Repeat this pose four times.

Third Block of Exercises: Build Lean Muscles

In this block, I won't name specific exercises, because weight-lifting exercises, especially for people above a certain age, have to be tailor-made. I might say pull-ups, push-ups, and dumbbell squats in negative and you may think, who can do these? Therefore, my advice is to consult with a personal trainer on which lean muscle-building weight-lifting exercises are the most fitting for you. Especially if you are a beginner weight lifter, I recommend having a professional around to avoid injuries. Don't get discouraged from doing weight-lifting exercises, since they are an essential form of workout for building lean muscles.

To gain lean muscle, you need to introduce weight training into your workout routine at least three times a week. Weight machines and free weights are both excellent ways to get maximum muscle gains. Remember, always consult with a personal trainer before you engage in any unfamiliar workout routine. I usually recommend starting weight-lifting workouts like squats, triceps overhead extensions, lunges, step-ups, deadlifts, and others with a single set of 10–12 repetitions. Start this single repetition with a weight that you can manage without being strained, but still being challenged a bit. The more you do the same workout, the better and stronger you'll become.

Gradually increase the repetitions within the sets, as well as the sets themselves. Let's say when you become comfortable with a weight, you could do three repetitions of sets with 12 reps in each.

When even these numbers of reps feel easy, you can increase the weight you're working with. The goal is to stay challenged all the time—without getting injured, of course. Your body will tell you when it's time to increase the weight. You should avoid getting comfortable with a weight, as there is no improvement in stagnation.

Try to follow a strict schedule with your weight workout; otherwise, you won't see visible progress. Keep the trainings consistent. It doesn't work if you skip a week and you try to do six weight workouts the next. As I said, you should be doing your strength training at least three times a week. You don't even have to do more, necessarily, because your muscles need a rest period between strength workouts to repair themselves and grow stronger. You can talk with your personal trainer about alternating upper and lower body workouts for better results.

This doesn't mean that you shouldn't train on the other days. On the days when you don't have weight training scheduled, you can do cardio workouts like walking, biking, and of course the stretching exercises presented in the first and second exercise blocks. As a matter of fact, you should also stretch after your weight workout to help your muscles become more flexible. Most trainings—and trainers—at gyms focus mainly on concentric movements, but by now we know that what you should be focusing on are mostly eccentric exercises.

Each weight-lifting exercise has a concentric and an eccentric part. For example, when you do biceps curls, lifting the weight is the concentric part of the exercise and releasing it is the eccentric. Most people focus on the lifting part and literally release the tension in their muscles when they bring the weight back to normal, dropping the weight. Not only does half of the muscle-building potential go unused, but dropping a larger weight like that can also cause injury. When you do strength workouts, focus on the negative. And slow down—it is a misconception that you have to do the repetitions as fast as a rabbit on speed.

Slowing down is one of the key features to build stronger muscles quickly.

Do a repetition in six seconds—let's say, where you do the concentric part in two seconds and the

89

eccentric in four. In other words, two counts to lift, four counts to lower the weight.

If you've started getting anxious because you're a 70-year-old lady who never went to the gym in her life, don't worry. First and foremost, it is never too late. Secondly, you don't have to do biceps sets with 40-pound weights. Start with one pound, or half a pound. Your aim is to keep your cells alive longer, not to be featured in the next *Pumping Iron* documentary. And let me tell you this: you'd be considered the most amazing person ever if you showed up at the gym, fully determined, doing your job. There's no shame in it. It's worthy of respect.

My daughter is 17 years old now and takes Zumba classes regularly. There she befriended a 68-year-old man named Leon. *Nomen est omen*, in his case—the man still looks like a lion. He trains every day with the same weights I do and goes to Zumba class after each of his weight trainings. He is 68 but doesn't look more than 50. And he is definitely stronger than many at the age of 40. My daughter told me when she is already out of breath during the class, Leon still jumps around like a teenager. He is amazing.

When I first met Leon, I asked him, "What keeps you so young?" You know what he told me? He said this:

"I work hard to exclude all negative energies around myself. I don't care what people think about me. They sometimes tell me I should be with one leg in the grave already instead of running on a treadmill. Why? Why should this be my fate at my age? I'm working hard to live in better physical and mental condition. Some might think I'm selfish, being so busy staying healthy. I should take my grandkids to the park instead of lifting weights. But you know what? This is exactly the reason why I keep myself busy at the gym every day: to stay strong and healthy to enjoy quality time at the playground with my grandkids.

"It matters what you think about yourself. You give that to the world. You can't give something you don't have. If you don't love yourself, you can't truly love others. If you don't take care of yourself, you won't be able to take real care of others, either. I love myself, and I love others. I know staying in shape largely contributes to my optimism. I also think that one should say thank you all the time. People are so rarely grateful. It pains me. Gratitude keeps you young. Being thankful will make you sweet instead of bitter. So thank you, sir, for listening!"

This is how he closed his sweet little monologue. God bless you, Leon.

Back to eccentric exercises—the concentric part of a biceps curl is when the muscle shortens in length, like in the lifting phase when you curl the weight toward your shoulder. The eccentric part is when you lower the weight back to the starting position. It is the lengthening phase. Your muscles need both of these types of exercise to get maximum results from your workout. Fitness experts have agreed that eccentric training is more important than concentric training because it induces muscle hypertrophy and thus lean muscle-building.

Slowing down the rep counts to six seconds has two major benefits. Firstly, it minimizes the probability of "cheating." When you do reps quickly, you strongly rely on momentum, and thus, you won't get maximum results out of your training. Secondly, if you do a repetition slower, your muscles will work more under tension. The more time your muscles spend under tension, the better your results—that's what studies have proved.

Consult with your physician or personal trainer about what exercises do they recommend for you.

Chapter 5: Anti-Aging Diet Principles

Experts say that to lose weight, nutrition has a bigger say than exercises—an exponentially bigger say, for that matter, in a 70:30% ratio. In other words, what you eat defines 70% of the outcome, while what you do is responsible for only 30%.

To improve aging effects, we saw how crucial, how essential, exercising is. However, exercises are just one part of aging prevention. Nutrition is the other key. This part of the book will focus on nutrition.

Just like exercising, the right diet is just as important for the maintenance of cellular defense systems, immunity, metabolism, and DNA repair. Previously in the book, we saw that proper cell repairing and replacement is essential to keep us energized, healthy, and young.

We require a healthy cellular defense system to keep us safe from environmental stresses like viruses, bacteria, fungi, and stressors-related aging. If we fail to defend our body against these stressors, we march directly into the arms of chronic diseases, premature aging, and other unpleasantries. Therefore, controlling and regulating our cellular defense systems is critical to having a good quality of life. Diet is considered a building block in maintaining cellular defenses.[xx]

We humans have five interlinked cellular defense systems: the immune system, the inflammatory response, redox regulation, metabolism, and DNA repair. These defense systems operate at a molecular level to combat various stressors to maintain the health of our physiology and reduce our risk of diseases.

Technological advances helped to prove that micronutrients have a strong link to cellular defense systems and therefore our overall health status. Vitamins, minerals, amino acids, fatty acids, and antioxidants play a crucial part in defense system maintenance. For example, antioxidant vitamins, like vitamins C and E, help in redox balance. [1] Vitamins are also linked to homeostatic regulation of cellular defenses linked to immunity, inflammation, and DNA repair.[xxi]

The reaction of the people when I confess my age amuses me a lot. They don't want to believe that I'm 50. They keep on asking what my secret is. Unfortunately, I don't have a cool story like radioactive spiders or kryptonite—it's all just exercise and healthy diet.

Eat Yourself to Live

Before you "learn to live" with a chronic condition, better try to prevent or reverse it. So what is the best anti-aging advice from a nutrition and lifestyle point of view to turn back the clock and maintain the life quality of your youth?

Sugar raises your insulin level, putting an unnatural demand on your body to process the energy you just consumed. Sugars, and simple carbohydrates in general, have an inflammatory effect on your body.

---

[1] Redox reactions control some cellular processes. For example, redox proteins must be collocated for redox regulation for the function of DNA in mitochondria. Vitamin C and E can help in that.

When you were younger, you could get away with a stomachache after carb-heavy meals, but with age, these foods backfire bitterly. Wrinkles will "invade" your face, you'll be sluggish, and as a consequence of lack of motion, your cells will start to atrophy and die. And so, the cocktail for aging will be ready. Do your present and future self a favor and ditch sugar, bread, cakes, pasta, potatoes, and porridge from your diet as much as you can.

Previously in this book, I explained exhaustively why exercise is essential in youth and health preservation. Exercising increases lean muscle mass. Certain types of food help increase lean muscle mass if paired with proper exercise. The best food for this purpose is mostly animal protein. Meats like poultry, beef, wild game, fish, and other seafood contain the greatest concentrations of essential and branched-chain amino acids. These meats also contain creatine, which is essential for building and maintaining lean muscle. Vegetarian readers, don't get discouraged—the essential amino acids and creatine you need to develop lean muscle mass can be bought in the form of dietary supplements, as well.

How much meat should you consume to get the amount of proteins, amino acids, and creatine you need on a daily basis? Some specialists say men should have a portion of meat 1.5 times bigger and thicker than their palm, and women should have a portion the same size and thickness of their palm.

I recommend keeping balance and variety regarding the meat you eat. Based on Subway and other fast food chains '"daily menu" idea, I developed my own "meat of the day" plan.

- Monday: beef
- Tuesday: shrimp, squids, or other type of seafood
- Wednesday: wild game meat (usually deer)
- Thursday: chicken
- Friday: salmon
- Saturday: chicken
- Sunday: no meat day

As you can see, I try to keep my meat consumption balanced. If one day I consume a heavier meat like beef, the next day I won't have game, but rather fish, a very light type of meat. There is a butchery close to our home, and I'm a regular customer there. Bill, the butcher, already knows what to prepare to me each time I go. I highly recommend buying your meat from a local butchery or farmers—a trustworthy and easily detectable source. I know it sounds troublesome to dig up a butcher and to buy so many types of meat and keep track of the meat's origin. However, this is the only body you have. It is up to you what lengths are you willing to go to keep it healthy.

Sometimes, when I know it will be busy a week, I preorder every type of meat at Bill's and pick up the entire weekly meat on Monday. I keep in my fridge the meat I'm going to eat on Monday and Tuesday and freeze the rest.

I buy the meat for my family, too, not only myself. I usually take my Igloo cooler to keep the large amount of meat I buy in a cold place all the time. Make sure all the meat you bought is fresh and was not frozen previously. Don't ever frost meat twice. Meat, once defrosted, has to be eaten within 24 hours.

Why is it so important to have a high protein intake for women?

Lean muscle mass doesn't help women in reducing mortality as it does men. However, a high protein intake is essential to maintain cognitive health.

So if lean muscle doesn't reduce mortality in women, why should they maintain a high protein intake? There are lots of reasons, but number one on the list is cognitive health. The *New England Journal of Medicine* discovered in a study performed on patients over the age of 65 that people with high blood sugar levels were at seven times greater risk of dementia.[xxii] As people get older, they are more and more inclined to reduce the effort they put into their nutrition. Many elderly people live on a "toast and tea" diet. This means that their main meals are toasts—pure carbs. They drink a lot of tea, which by itself is not unhealthy, but suppresses appetite. If they put processed sugar into the tea, that's even worse. The high-carb diet they consume damages their brain cells, leading to cognitive decline and ultimately dementia. To overcome this problem— to restore the optimal blood sugar and keep the brain safe—new diet patterns have to be adopted. High vegetable, lean meat, and healthy fat consumption can turn things around.

Bad habits die hard. However, American-style breakfasts are not your friend in youth preservation. Toasts, sugary cereals, and artificial orange juice gained from concentrate should be avoided. If you crave a fresh juice in the morning, squeeze it yourself. Are fruits expensive? Well, medications are even pricier. Don't save five bucks today just to be forced to spend 500 tomorrow.

Some dietitians warn against eating eggs in the morning because it might raise cholesterol levels. I don't agree with this deterrence. Low cholesterol levels are associated with dementia, as a matter of fact. Low cholesterol levels can be just as harmful as high ones. Eating two to three eggs in the morning is actually very good for your body. Eggs are rich in protein, and morning protein intake is very beneficial to jumpstart your body.[xxiii]

Your body has its own cholesterol-making machine. In other words, the cholesterol you eat will raise your cholesterol, but some food enhances your cholesterol-making machine's activity too. These elements are mostly saturated and trans fats. Eggs, for that matter, have a very low level of saturated fat. One large egg contains about 1.5 grams of saturated fat, which is a fraction of the amount of saturated fat in a tablespoon of butter you might cook that egg in.[xxiv] No butter or oil, nonstick pan, and more eggs—the solution for a low-cholesterol breakfast.

Keep Your Spirits High

As people grow older, in many cases they lose their motivation to do things. They convince themselves that they are old, that certain activities are not for them, and that they shouldn't even try doing it. Research suggests that low testosterone, vitamin D, omega-3, and high blood sugars and insulin can be the cause of low moods. Average American people have a diet rich in simple carbs and processed food that can cause insulin dysfunction, which has an inflammatory effect and results in weight gain.

How do you avoid mood decline and all the other negative byproducts of a high-carb diet? Exercise combined with low-carb diet. From as little exercise as walking for 20–30 minutes, to stretching or weight lifting, you can improve your blood pressure and improve your overall mood and health. Vegetables and fruits have an alkalinizing effect. Balancing alkali and acid in your body and maintaining a healthy pH is essential for your well-being.

To understand your body's alkali needs, know that water has a neutral pH level of seven. Your blood, in normal conditions, has a pH of 7.35–7.45; therefore, it is slightly alkaline. Our body fights hard every day to maintain our healthy pH. The more acidic food you consume, the harder this job will be for your body. Vegetables and fruits are considered to be alkaline in nature. Even citruses, which have an acidic pH, when metabolized, leave an alkaline residue.[xxv]

Fruits and vegetables provide a good amount of minerals, antioxidants, and essential vitamins that help the immune system, protect DNA from damage, and fight cancers. They also maintain heart health and promote optimal health. Do not let the intake of essential proteins and vegetables decline in your diet as you age. You need them more than ever. Believe it or not, age is just a mental state, not a judgment that can't be avoided. Don't limit your mind and body with your thoughts. Eat clean and move every day, and keep your years for the calendar, not the mirror.

The human body needs much more potassium than sodium. The typical U.S. diet, unfortunately, is quite the opposite. Americans average about 3300 milligrams of sodium per day, about 75% of which comes from processed foods, while only getting about 2900 milligrams of potassium daily. Sodium and potassium have opposite effects on heart health. High salt intake increases blood pressure, which can lead to heart disease, while high potassium intake can help relax blood vessels and excrete sodium and decrease blood pressure.[xxvi]

What about grains, starches, and other "evils"?

Whole grains, legumes, and many low-fat dairy products are excellent sources of nutrition, like dietary fiber, proteins, vitamins, and minerals. These foods are beneficial and healthy when they are not overeaten. They contribute to a balanced, healthy diet, except for individuals who, due to allergy or digestion difficulties, can't eat them.

I'm a true advocate of variety in nutrition. Each

food contributes something unique for the body to utilize. Therefore, I always recommend not excluding all whole grains, legumes, and dairy products from your diet unless it is necessary. However, you should reduce their consumption as much as possible. I have a whole grain pastry on Sundays, my cheat day.

Sweet potatoes are an excellent source of vitamin A. Studies show they help reduce the number of fat cells. [xxvii] They have a healthy number of numerous vitamins and minerals, including potassium. While they are high in carbs, there are times when it is advantageous to increase carbs. They are also sweet and satisfying and have a low GI rating. I recommend the occasional and moderate consumption of sweet potatoes as long as the total daily carb consumption doesn't exceed the recommended level.

Chapter 6: The Best Anti-Aging Foods—And the Worst

In this chapter, I will tell you what the best anti-aging foods are. I will also give you a sample weekly diet plan where I mix the best knowledge I got from dieticians with my own experience.

Best Foods for Anti-Aging

We know that having healthy skin with as few wrinkles as possible is not only a question of nutrition, but also getting enough sleep, using sunscreen, drinking sufficient water, and exercising. Above all these comes nutrition.

Recommended carbs: The best rest you can give to your skin is to consume low-glycemic carbs (like oats) and avoid high-glycemic carbs (like refined bread, pasta, and white rice). High-glycemic foods are the cause of acne and, later on, wrinkles.

Recommended fats: Macadamia nut oil, olive oil, and avocado. When it comes to fat, the more monounsaturated, the better. This type of fat helps retain your skin's hydration and helps the absorption of more nutrients and vitamins. Olive oil is high in omega-3, which improves circulation and gives the skin rosy glow. It also contains polyphenols that may help prevent age-related diseases.

Recommended proteins: Lean meat like beef sirloin is rich in high-quality protein. It is essential in collagen building. Chicken, fish, seafood, and eggs are also rich in protein and therefore very helpful in retaining your younger self.

Recommended vitamins: Pink grapefruits, oranges, and parsley are loaded with vitamin C. This vitamin helps create collagen, which is a subdermal connective tissue that makes skin look smooth and stay flexible. Oranges and grapefruits are rich in water, and therefore, they serve as hydration sources, as well. Brussels sprouts are also high in vitamins C and A, having lots of skin benefits. Pomegranate juice and pomegranate seeds contain ellagic acid and punicalagin. Ellagic is a polyphenol compound that fights damage from free radicals. Punicalagin is a super-nutrient that is suggested to increase your body's collagen-preserving capacity.

Recommended omega-3 source: Cold-water fish such as salmon, mackerel, and sardines are rich in omega-3 fats. Some specialists suggest that omega-3 can keep skin cancer cells from spreading. Chia seed and flax seed are also rich in omega-3 fatty acid and furthermore in dietary fiber and antioxidants. I use chia and flax seeds in my diet, adding a small spoonful of each to my morning meals.

Recommended liquid: Water and the right amount of it. As we become older, we feel less and less thirsty; therefore, we drink less water and can become chronically dehydrated. The human body is mostly water. Imagine how your cells look if you're dehydrated. You'll feel exhausted, and your energy levels and cognitive functions will drop.

Recommended berries: Although you can't go wrong with any berry, blueberries contain the most antioxidants and nutrients among them. Compounds in blueberries (and other berries) alleviate oxidative damage and inflammation. These problems are associated with age-related deficits, like memory and motor function. Blueberries can give extra protection against skin-damaging free radicals coming from sun exposure and stress.

Recommended alcohol: Wine. Red wine in moderation can protect against heart disease, diabetes, and age-related memory loss. Based on current research, red wine proves the most beneficial results since it contains resveratrol, a compound that is likely to activate genes that slow cellular aging (according to animal-based studies).[xxviii]

Recommended firming foods: Spinach and kale. These two vegetables contain a lot of phytonutrients (antioxidant compounds) that protect you against damage caused by the sun. Spinach is rich in beta-carotene and lutein, two nutrients that have been shown to improve skin elasticity. Why do you think Popeye's forearm could stretch like that? Tomatoes are also a good choice for firming, thanks to the lycopene they contain. Lycopene is responsible for the pigment that gives them their rich red color. Eating tomatoes may parry UV-induced damage like wrinkles.

Recommended brown-spot fighting drink: Green tea. This simple drink is rich in catechins and polyphenols. The first is one of the most effective compounds for preventing hyperpigmentation, a typical problem of those who are often exposed to the sun. The second are antioxidants that combat free-radical damage. Also, they can reverse the effects of aging.

Recommended fruits for hydration: Watermelon. Loaded with vitamin C, lycopene, and potassium, the watermelon is a super-fruit that helps to regulate the balance of water and nutrients in cells. It is also one of the best desserts in summer. Try cooling it off before eating it.

Recommended food to fight heart disease: Garlic is said to slow the hardening of the arteries, therefore preventing heart disease and strokes. It can also help fight inflammation and cartilage damage due to arthritis.

Avoid These Foods

Sugar and High-Fructose Corn Syrup

Where can you find them? In table sugar (white and brown), soft drinks, fruit juices, candies, bakery products, ice cream, and in many more foods.

Why are they unhealthy? Well, where should I start this long list of reasons? First of all, sugars are empty carbs. They have no nutritional value. They contain no protein, no healthy fats, no nutrients, no enzymes. They just pull minerals out of your body during digestion. Not to mention the crazy number of calories they inject into our bodies. Sugar calories create a kind of hormone frenzy when eaten, but as soon as its effect is gone, we'll crave more.[xxix]

Dairy Products

Where can you find them? In products like milk, cheese, butter, cottage cheese, or yogurts. The low-fat versions of these products are especially harmful.

Why are they unhealthy? One of the greatest arguments against dairy consumption is that is "unnatural." After all, we are the only species that consumes milk after we drop out of diapers and the only one that consumes the milk of species other than our own (like cows, goats, etc.). While in some cultures, dairy consumption was never a thing (for example, many Asian people and Native Americans can't digest dairy), after the agricultural revolution, some cultures adopted dairy consumption—for example, in Northern Europe. Lactose intolerance (lactose is milk sugar, the main carbohydrate of dairy products) affects 75% of the population, even today.

My objection against dairy products is because the dairy products we can access day by day at the supermarket are not healthy ones. Processed dairy products lose almost all of their natural nutritional value. For example, only a cup of whole milk coming from a grass-fed cow contains calcium (276 mg, 28% of the RDA - Recommended Daily Allowance), Vitamin D (24% of the RDA), riboflavin (B2) (26% of the RDA), vitamin B12 (18% of the RDA), potassium (10% of the RDA), phosphorus (22% of the RDA), and some vitamin A, B1, B6, selenium, zinc, and magnesium.[xxx]

113

Whole milk is quite nutritious. If you are lactose tolerant and can access non-processed milk, I recommend the consumption of it. However, keep in mind that not all dairy products have the same nutritional value, even more so when we think about their processed version. Long story short—consume non-processed, non-low-fat, whole dairy products only.

Vegetable Oils

Where can you find them? Sunflower oil, cottonseed oil, soybean oil, safflower oil, corn oil, rapeseed oil, and others.

Why are they unhealthy? Vegetable oils are technically some of the newest foods on our plate. People in the 19th century didn't even know what they were. We started producing and consuming them only in the 20th century. But since then, we consume them like water. Well, almost like that. The average American vegetable oil consumption is 70 pounds per person per year.

Vegetable oils contain high levels of polyunsaturated fats, also called PUFAs. Previously, I talked about monounsaturated fat and its benefits. The human body's fat content is about 97% saturated and monounsaturated fat. Fat is necessary for rebuilding cells and stable hormone production. However, polyunsaturated fats are very unstable and oxidize easily, causing inflammation and mutation in cells. This process is the bed of many severe illnesses, from cancer to heart disease.[xxxi]

Trans Fats

Where can you find them? They are mentioned as "hydrogenated" or "partially hydrogenated" oils and can be found in margarine and many other processed foods.

Why are they unhealthy? These hydrogenated fats are created through a very disgusting process that involves pumping hydrogen molecules into vegetable oil. This process changes their chemical structure, turning the oil from liquid to solid—and giving them an extra-long lifetime. Studies and clinical research showed that trans fats significantly increase the risk of heart disease, diabetes, metabolic syndrome, arthritis, and many more afflictions.[xxxii]

Artificial Sweeteners

Where can you find them? Aspartame, sucralose, cyclamates, saccharin, and acesulfame.

Why are they unhealthy? A study at the Multiethnic Study of Atherosclerosis showed that daily diet drink consumption could be correlated with a 67% greater risk for type 2 diabetes and 36% greater risk for metabolic syndrome. Sweeteners don't necessarily save you from those extra calories, either. Researchers proved sweeteners "may prevent us from associating sweetness with caloric intake. As a result, we may crave more sweets, tend to choose sweet food over nutritious food, and gain weight."[xxxiii]

Weekly Sample Menu

Monday

Detox drink of the day: Strawberry-lime water

- 1 cup strawberries
- 1 lime
- 10 mint leaves

Prepare the drink a night before. Into a large pitcher mix 2 L (64 oz.) of water, one cup of sliced strawberries, and one sliced lime. Optionally you can add 10 mint leaves as well. Mix them thoroughly and cover the pitcher for the night. Drink this healthy juice the next day.

Breakfast: Blueberry smoothie

- 1 cup (240 milliliters) coconut, almond or whole milk or water
- 1 ½ cups (210 grams) blueberries, fresh or frozen

- 2 medium cold or frozen ripe bananas
- 1 tbsp. lemon juice (plus-minus to taste)
- 1 tsp. lemon zest
- 1 tsp. vanilla extract

Blend everything together in a blender until well combined. If you wish, you can add one scoop of vanilla-flavored protein powder to boost your morning protein intake.

Lunch: Lemon rosemary chicken (two servings)

- 2 ½ lbs boneless, skinless chicken breast
- 4 cloves garlic, crushed
- 4 tbsp. fresh rosemary leaves, strip the leaves from the stem
- 3 tbsp. of olive oil
- 1 ½ lemons' zest and juice
- Himalayan salt and pepper to taste (try to reduce the amount of salt as much as possible)

Preparation: Preheat the oven to 450 degrees Fahrenheit. Put sliced chicken on a baking plate. Season and coat the chicken with the garlic, salt, pepper, rosemary leaves, and lemon zest and drizzle it with olive oil. Roast it for 20 minutes in the oven. Add the lemon juice to the baking pan, drizzling the chicken with it. Roast for five more minutes. Remove the chicken from the baking sheet and coat it with the pan juices. Garnish it with garden salad mix.

Dinner: Oven-roasted garlic cabbage

- 1 big green cabbage cut into 1-inch slices
- 5 cloves of minced garlic
- 3 tbsp. of olive oil
- Himalayan salt and freshly ground pepper to taste

Preparation: Preheat the oven to 400 degrees Fahrenheit. Coat both sides of the cabbage with the garlic, salt, pepper, and olive oil. Roast one side of the cabbage for 20 minutes, then flip them and roast the other side as well for 10–15 minutes.

Tuesday

Detox drink of the day: Raspberry-mint water

- 1 cup raspberries
- 10 mint leaves
- 1 lime

Prepare the drink a night before. Into a large pitcher mix 2 L (64 oz.) of water, one cup of raspberries, and one sliced lime. Add five mint leaves as well. Mix them thoroughly and cover the pitcher for the night. Drink this healthy juice the next day.

Breakfast: Vanilla-blueberry smoothie

- 1-inch peeled ginger
- ½ cup of frozen or fresh blueberries
- 2 handfuls of baby spinach
- 1 scoop of vanilla powder
- A few ice cubes
- 10 ounces of full-fat coconut milk (unsweetened)

Blend everything together in a blender until well combined.

Lunch: Salmon with citrus salad (two servings)

- ¾ lb salmon filets
- ½ tsp. Himalayan salt
- ¼ tsp. freshly ground pepper
- ½ lb mixed greens
- 1 cup sugar snap peas
- 1 radish, thinly sliced
- 1/3 cup roasted sunflower seeds
- Juice of ½ orange and ½ lemon
- 1 tbsp. olive oil

Preheat the oven to 425 degrees Fahrenheit. Season both sides of the salmon. Add one teaspoon of olive oil to a nonstick pan and on medium heat fry the salmon skin-side up for 2–3 minutes until nice and crispy. Then put them on a baking pan (covered with a baking sheet) and insert them into the oven. Bake it until salmon feels cooked through. (A fresh salmon needs 15 minutes; a frozen one needs 30 minutes.) While the salmon cooks, combine the vegetables in a large bowl with the juices and season the mixture to taste.

Dinner: Cantaloupe with avocado salad (four servings)

- 3 tbsp. of freshly squeezed lime juice
- 4 tsp. of raw honey
- 2 tbsp. of olive oil
- ½ tsp. Himalayan salt
- 1 cantaloupe (3 lbs) seeded and quartered.
- 1 avocado
- 1 cup of cherry tomatoes, halved

Mix the lime juice, olive oil, honey, and salt in a large bowl. Halve the cantaloupe quarters lengthwise and peel their skin. Slice them lengthwise into half-inch pieces. Dice the avocado half-inch thick. Add the avocado and cantaloupe into the bowl and coat them with the mixture.

Wednesday

Detox drink of the day: Rose-lime water

- Rose extract or the petals of two bids of red roses
- 1 lime

Prepare the drink a night before. Into a large pitcher mix 2 L (64 oz.) of water, add the petals of two scarlet red roses or a few drops of rose extract and one sliced lime. Add five mint leaves if you wish. Mix them thoroughly and cover the pitcher for the night. Drink this healthy juice the next day.

Breakfast: Granola mixture

- 1 cup of cashews
- ¾ cup of almonds
- ¼ cup shelled pumpkin seeds
- ¼ cup shelled sunflower seeds
- ½ cup unsweetened coconut flakes
- ¼ cup coconut oil
- 1 tsp. vanilla extract
- A little stevia to taste
- A little Himalayan salt to taste

Preparation: Preheat the oven for 300 degrees Fahrenheit. Mix the cashews, almonds, pumpkin and sunflower seeds, and coconut flakes into a blender and break them into smaller pieces. In a small pot melt together the coconut oil, vanilla, and stevia. Add the blended mixture to the coconut oil pot and mix everything together. Spread the mixture on a baking sheet and cook it for 20 minutes. When the mixture is lightly browned, remove it from heat and cool it off.

Lunch: Cuban picadillo lettuce wraps[xxxiv]

For the picadillo
- 1 lb ground beef, preferably grass-fed
- 2 tbsp. tallow, lard, or coconut oil
- 1 medium onion, about 1.5 cups diced small
- 1 large green bell pepper, about 1.5 cups diced
- ½ tsp. salt
- 1 tsp. black pepper, freshly ground
- 1 tsp. ground cumin
- ½ tsp. ground cinnamon
- 1 14 oz. can whole tomatoes
- ¼ cup currants
- 2 tbsp. green olives with pimiento, diced

- 2 tbsp. drained capers
- 2 tbsp. olive brine (or white wine vinegar and salt to taste)

For the pico de gallo
- ⅓ cup minced shallot or red onion
- ⅔ cup diced tomatoes
- 2 tbsp. minced cilantro
- 2 tsp. fresh lime juice
- Salt to taste

To serve
- Lettuce leaves or cabbage leaves
- Cooked brown or white rice (optional)
- Chopped cilantro (optional)

Heat large skillet or Dutch oven over medium heat. Add beef. Crumble and stir occasionally as it cooks. Remove and set aside. Add tallow or oil to a pan. Add onions and cook until beginning to soften about 3–4 minutes. Add bell pepper and cook for three more minutes. Stir in garlic, then add the salt, black pepper, cumin, and cinnamon and stir for 30 seconds, until fragrant.

Add cooked beef, canned tomatoes, currants, diced olives, capers, and olive brine. Break up the

tomatoes into small pieces while the mixture comes to a boil.
Reduce heat to low, cover, and simmer for 10–20 minutes.

Meanwhile, prepare the pico de gallo. Combine minced shallot, chopped tomatoes, minced cilantro, lime juice, and a dash of salt, then set aside.

To serve, fill each lettuce leaf with the beef mixture, a spoonful of rice (if desired), and a spoonful of pico de gallo or cilantro.

Dinner: Raspberry smoothie

- 1 ½ cups unsweetened almond milk (or water)
- ¼ cups chia seed
- ½ cup frozen raspberries
- 2 tsp. raw almond butter (optional)
- 2 handfuls of spinach
- 5 mint leaves

Mix everything together until nice and smooth.

Note: You can switch the breakfast and the dinner at this meal.

Thursday

Detox drink of the day: Mint-lime water

- 10 mint leaves
- 1 lime

Prepare the drink a night before. Into a large pitcher mix 2 L (64 oz.) of water, 10 mint leaves, and one sliced lime. Mix them thoroughly and cover the pitcher for the night. Drink this healthy juice the next day.

Breakfast: Apple breakie

- 2 cups of raw walnuts
- 1 cup of macadamia nuts
- 2 apples, peeled and diced (I recommend pink lady apples)
- 1 tbsp. coconut oil
- 1 tbsp. ground cinnamon
- 2 cups of almond milk or water
- 1 14 oz. full fat coconut milk

In a food processor ground the walnuts and macadamia nuts until smoothened. Sauté the apples in coconut oil for five minutes in a medium bowl. Then add the smoothened nut mix and cinnamon to the bowl, stirring constantly cook it for a minute. Add the coconut milk and almond milk to the mixture, reduce heat and stirring occasionally let the mixture cook for 25 minutes.

Lunch: Cajun garlic shrimp noodles

- 3 cloves garlic, crushed
- 3 tbsp. grass-fed butter
- 10–20 jumbo shrimps, detailed

Cajun seasoning

- 1 Tsp. paprika
- Dash cayenne
- ½ tsp. Himalayan sea salt
- Dash red pepper flakes
- 1 Tsp. garlic granules
- 1 Tsp. onion powder

Other

- 2 large zucchinis, spiraled
- Red pepper, sliced
- Onion, sliced
- 1 Tbsp. grass-fed cow butter

Spiral your zucchini using a spiralizer, then set aside. Combine Cajun seasoning in a bowl and toss with shrimp. Heat butter and garlic in a nonstick pan. Add in red pepper and onion and sauté for 3–4 minutes. Add in Cajun shrimp and let cook until opaque.

In a separate pan heat the remaining butter and lightly sauté zucchini noodles for three minutes. Place zucchini noodles in a bowl and top with garlic Cajun shrimp and veggie mixture. Taste and add salt and seasoning as desired.[xxxv]

Dinner: Chicken avocado salad (two servings)

- 6 oz. pasture chicken breasts cooked
- 1 avocado, peeled and sliced
- ¼ cup chopped onion
- 4 cups baby spinach

Halve the amount of spinach, avocado, chicken, and onion and lay them onto two separate plates. Drizzle it with apple cider vinegar and olive oil. Add salt and pepper to taste.

Friday

Detox drink of the day: Blackberry-lemon water

- 1 cup blackberry
- 1 lemon

Prepare the drink a night before. Into a large pitcher mix 2 L (64 oz.) of water, one cup of blackberries, and one sliced lemon. Mix them thoroughly and cover the pitcher for the night. Drink this healthy juice the next day.

Breakfast: Omelet muffins (for eight muffins)

- 8 eggs
- 8 oz. cooked ham
- 1 cup diced onion
- 1 cup diced bell pepper
- Salt and pepper to taste
- 2 tbsp. of water

Preheat the oven to 350 degrees Fahrenheit. Grease eight muffin papers with coconut oil. Mix all the ingredients together in a large bowl and add them to the muffin papers. Bake them for 20 minutes.

Lunch: The bowl of doom[xxxvi]

- 3 sweet potatoes
- 1 lb. ground beef
- 5 green onions
- 1 large avocado
- 2 eggs
- Salsa
- 1 tbsp. cumin
- Salt/pepper
- Olive oil
- Coconut oil

Preparing the bowl of doom

Start with peeling and dicing your sweet potatoes. The smaller you cut them the quicker they cook. Once they're diced, heat a skillet or wok over medium-high heat. Add a spoonful of coconut oil into the pan and when it's melted, add the sweet potatoes. Season it with salt to taste. Cook them until they've softened a bit, stirring frequently.

Transfer the cooked sweet potato to a bowl, and then use the leftover oil to brown your ground beef. Season the beef with the cumin, Himalayan salt, and 2 teaspoons of garlic powder.

While the beef is cooking, chop your green onions. Also, heat up another pan to make the eggs.

Once the beef is browned, add your green onions to the pan and cook for a couple more minutes. Then add your sweet potato cubes. Cook it until you start seeing the beef get a little bit crispy (not too crispy).

Cook as many eggs as many dishes you're preparing however you like: omelet, scrambled eggs, or regular fried eggs.

Halve the avocado, peel it, and slice it. Finally, put some salsa in a little cup and design your bowl of doom plate.

Dinner: colorful salad

- 1 lettuce

- 1 large avocado
- 2 handfuls of cherry tomatoes
- ½ cucumber
- Handful of coriander (cilantro)
- 4 rashers of bacon
- Half a handful of feta cheese (optional but tastier)
- Mustard
- Extra virgin olive oil
- Balsamic vinegar
- 1 lemon

In a medium nonstick pan cook the bacon until it's crispy. While it's sizzling away, chop the other ingredients into half-inch cubes. Mix everything in a bowl. When the bacon is done, chop it into thin slices and add it to the veggies. Drizzle the salad with the feta cheese.

Pour about two shot glasses of extra virgin olive oil into a cup and add a shot of balsamic vinegar, a tablespoon of mustard, the juice of the lemon, and a pinch of Himalayan salt. Drizzle the mixture over the salad.

Saturday

Detox drink of the day: Grapefruit-mint water

- 10 mint leaves
- 1 grapefruit, sliced

Prepare the drink a night before. Into a large pitcher mix 2 L (64 oz.) of water, the grapefruit, and 10 mint leaves. Mix them thoroughly and cover the pitcher for the night. Drink this healthy juice the next day.

Breakfast: strawberry pancakes

- 1 ½ cups of almond meal
- 2 eggs
- ½ tsp. vanilla extract
- ½ tsp. ground cinnamon
- ½ cup applesauce
- ¼ tsp. baking powder
- ¼ cup coconut milk (full fat, unsweetened) or water
- 1 tsp. olive oil
- 1 cup fresh or frozen strawberries

In a bowl combine the almond meal, vanilla extract, cinnamon, eggs, baking powder, and coconut milk (or water). In a nonstick pan spread the olive oil. When the oil is hot, add the batter to the pan and fry it on one side for a few minutes. Avoid burning. Then flip the pancake and fry it on the other side, too. Repeat this step until the batter is gone. In a food processor puree the strawberries and add them to the pancakes.

Lunch: Tuna salad

- 1 avocado
- 1 lemon juiced, to taste
- 1 tbsp. chopped onion to taste
- 5 ounces cooked or canned wild tuna
- Himalayan salt to taste
- Fresh ground pepper to taste

Halve the avocado without peeling it. Scoop the middle of both avocado halves into a bowl, leaving a quarter-inch thick layer of avocado on each half.
Add the lemon juice and the onion to the scooped avocado in the bowl and mix them together. Add the tuna, salt, and pepper, and combine them

thoroughly. Taste and adjust if needed. Fill the avocado halves with the tuna salad.

Dinner: Salmon salad (you can use chicken instead of salmon)

- 4 ounces grilled or baked salmon
- 3–4 cup seasonal greens
- ½ cup sliced zucchini and squash
- ½ cup raspberries
- 1 tbsp. balsamic glaze
- 2 tbsp. avocado or olive oil
- Salt and pepper
- 2 thyme sprigs
- Parmesan crumbles (optional)
- Lemon juice

Preheat the oven to 450 degrees Fahrenheit. Season the salmon with salt and pepper to taste. Put it on a baking sheet and drizzle it with olive oil. Cook it for 10–15 minutes depending on the thickness of the salmon slice.

Slice your zucchini and squash, and sauté in skillet with ½ tablespoon oil and a little bit of pepper and salt. Once the zucchini and salmon are cooked, build your bowl. Drizzle it with balsamic glaze, thyme sprigs leaves, and the rest of your oil. Mix everything together and place in a bowl. Add the raspberries last with a touch of lemon juice on top. Sprinkle it with parmesan if desired.

Sunday (attention: some preparation for lunch should be made in the morning)

Detox drink of the day: Pomegranate-mint water

- 10 mint leaves
- 1 cup of pomegranate seeds

Prepare the drink a night before. Into a large pitcher mix 2 L (64 oz.) of water, one cup of pomegranate, and 10 mint leaves. Mix them thoroughly and cover the pitcher for the night. Drink this healthy juice the next day.

Breakfast: Apple cinnamon smoothie

- 10 oz. unsweetened almond milk
- ½ avocado
- 1 apple, peeled and diced
- 1 scoop of vanilla protein
- 1 tsp. of peeled and minced ginger
- 1 tsp. cinnamon

Blend everything together in a blender until smooth.

Lunch: Broccoli salad with cashew cream

For the dressing:
- ¾ cup roasted, salted cashews (105 g)
- 5 ½ tbsp. water
- 1 tbsp. apple cider vinegar
- 4 tsp. yellow curry powder
- 2 ½ tsp. light agave
- ½ tsp. salt
- Pinch of pepper

For the salad:

- 4 cups broccoli, cut into bite-sized pieces
- ¼ cup red onion, diced
- ½ cup cilantro, roughly chopped
- ¼ cup dried cranberries, roughly chopped
- 2 tbsp. sunflower seeds
- 2 tbsp. roasted, salted cashews roughly chopped

Put the cashews in a bowl and pour water over it until covered. Refrigerate the bowl for five hours. After that put the cashews into a food processor. Add the remaining dressing ingredients to the cashews and blend until smooth. Set it aside.

In a bigger bowl mix the broccoli, cilantro, red onions, and cranberries. Stir them until they are even and let them "rest" for about an hour. Before serving, add the sunflower seeds and cashews and mix them.[xxxvii]

Dinner: Spaghetti squash bake

- 1 spaghetti squash
- 1 tsp. extra-virgin olive oil
- 1 clove garlic, crushed
- 3 handfuls fresh spinach
- 1 cup tomato sauce of choice
- 1 egg
- 1 ½ tbsp. Italian seasoning, more to taste
- ½ tsp. red pepper flakes, more to taste
- 1 tbsp. garlic powder
- ½ tsp. freshly ground pepper
- ½ tsp. salt
- ¼ cup fresh parmesan cheese (optional)

Preheat the oven to 375 degrees Fahrenheit.

Cut spaghetti squash in half and scoop out seeds. Drizzle with olive oil, sea salt, and black pepper. Line the baking sheet with parchment paper. Lay spaghetti squash facedown on the baking sheet and add ¼ cup water. Bake for about 30 minutes until fork tender. Let it cool.

Once cool, scrape out spaghetti squash using a fork and place in a medium mixing bowl and set aside. In a small skillet over medium heat, heat oil and sauté garlic. Add spinach and sauté until wilted. Add spinach and garlic mixture, shredded chicken, tomato sauce, egg, cheese if using, and spices to the bowl with the spaghetti squash. Mix until well combined.

Transfer entire mixture to a baking dish. Sprinkle with fresh Parmesan and red pepper flakes. Bake at 375 degrees Fahrenheit for 10 minutes. Broil on high for 3–5 minutes or until the cheese has started to bubble and brown."[xxxviii]

References

Academy. Khan. *"Cellular Respiration."* Khan Academy.
https://www.khanacademy.org/science/biolog y/cellular-respiration-and-fermentation

Alleva R, Di Donato F, Strafella E, Staffolani S, Nocchi L, Borghi B, Pignotti E, Santarelli L, Tomasetti M. *"Effect of ascorbic acid-rich diet on in vivo-induced oxidative stress."* Br J Nutr. 2011;Sep 16:1–10.

A. R. Brooks-Wilson. *„Genetics of healthy aging and longevity".* Human Genetics. 2013. 132 Issue 12, pp. 1323-38

Campellone. Joseph V. *"Muscle Atrophy."* Mediline Plus. 2016.
https://medlineplus.gov/ency/article/003188. htm

Chan. James. *"Strength Training For Fat Loss: Building A Bigger Engine!"* Body Building. 2016.
https://www.bodybuilding.com/content/stren

gth-training-for-fat-loss-building-a-bigger-engine.html

Crane P. et al. *"Glucose Levels and Risk of Dementia."* NEJM. Sept 2013. Vol 369. National Hospital Discharge Survey (NHDS), National Center for Health Statistics.

Daily. Science. *"Toba Catastrophe Theory."*
Science Daily.
https://www.sciencedaily.com/terms/toba_catastrophe_theory.htm

Diven, Alison. *"Cuban Picadillo Lettuce wraps."*
The Nourishing Gourmet. 2014.
http://www.thenourishinggourmet.com/2014/07/cuban-picadillo-lettuce-wraps-gf-df-paleo-friendly.html

Drew. Janice E. *"Cellular Defense System Gene Expression Profiling of Human Whole Blood: Opportunities to Predict Health Benefits in Response to Diet."* Advances in Nutrition. 2012.
http://advances.nutrition.org/content/3/4/499.full

Dr. Axe. *"Is Sugar Bad for You? Here's How It Destroys Your Body."* Dr. Axe – Food is Medicine. 2018. https://draxe.com/is-sugar-bad-for-you/

Dr. Mercola. *"To Protect Your Heart, Your Sodium to Potassium Ratio Is More Important Than Your Overall Salt Intake."* Mercola. 2014. http://articles.mercola.com/sites/articles/archive/2014/08/25/sodium-potassium-ratio.aspx

Esmonde-White. Miranda. *"Aging Backwards."* Harper Wave. 2014

Gangemi, Stephen. *"Elevate Your Cholesterol Profile, Elevate Your Health."* Dr. Gangemi. 2018. http://www.drgangemi.com/health-articles/diet-nutrition/elevate-cholesterol-elevate-health/

Gunnars, Kris. *"Is Dairy Bad Or Good?"* Authority Nutrition. 2017. https://authoritynutrition.com/is-dairy-bad-or-good/

Hötting K., Röder B. *"Beneficial effects of physical exercise on neuroplasticity and cognition."* US National Library of Medicine National Institutes of Health. 2013. https://www.ncbi.nlm.nih.gov/pubmed/23623982

Hummusapien. *"The Best Vegan Broccoli Salad."* Hummusapien. 2016. https://www.hummusapien.com/vegan-broccoli-salad/

Lexi. *"Cajun Garlic Shrimp Noodle Bowls."* Lexi's Clean Kitchen. 2014. http://lexiscleankitchen.com/2014/09/08/cajun-garlic-shrimp-noodle-bowls/

Lexi. *"Italian Style Spaghetti Squash Bake."* Lexi's Clean Kitchen. 2013. http://lexiscleankitchen.com/2013/05/25/italian-style-spaghetti-squash-bake/

Light. Cooking. *"10 Nutrition Myths."* Cooking Light. 2016. http://www.cookinglight.com/eating-smart/nutrition-101/nutrition-myths-facts/eggs-cholesterol-levels

Mann, Denise. *"Trans Fats: The Science and the Risks."* WebMD. 2018. https://www.webmd.com/diet/features/trans-fats-science-and-risks#1

Med-Health. *"Benefits of Muscular Strength."* Med-Health. 2017. http://www.med-health.net/Benefits-Of-Muscular-Strength.html

Picture I. Surekha. *„Human Cell – Properties, Diagram, Parts, Pictures, Structure."* Diseases Pictures. 2016. http://diseasespictures.com/human-cell-functions-diagram-parts-pictures-structure/

Picture 2. Wallance, Michael. M.D. "*The Digestive System & How it Works.*" National Institute of Diabetes and Digestive and Kidney Diseases. 2013. https://www.niddk.nih.gov/health-information/digestive-diseases/digestive-system-how-it-works

R. E. Van Pelt, F. A. Dinneno, D. R. Seals, and P. P. Jones. "*Age-related decline in RMR in physically active men: relation to exercise volume and energy intake.*" Am J Physiol Endocrinol Metab, PubMed PMID: 11500320. 2001.

Schaefer, Anna. "*Red Wine and Type 2 Diabetes: Is There a Link?*" Health Line. 2017. https://www.healthline.com/health/diabetes/red-wine-and-type-2-diabetes#1

S. M. Jeyakumar, A. Vajreswari, B. Sesikeran, and N. V. Giridharan, "*Vitamin A Supplementation Induces Adipose Tissue Loss through Apoptosis in Lean but Not in Obese Rats of the WNIN/OB Strain.*" Journal of Molecular Endocrinology. 2005. http://jme.endocrinology-journals.org/content/35/2/391.full

Strawbridge, Holly. "*Artificial sweeteners: sugar-free, but at what cost?*" Harvard Health

Publications. 2012. http://www.health.harvard.edu/blog/artificial-sweeteners-sugar-free-but-at-what-cost-201207165030

Surekha. „*Human Cell – Properties, Diagram, Parts, Pictures, Structure.*" Diseases Pictures. 2016. http://diseasespictures.com/human-cell-functions-diagram-parts-pictures-structure/

Tan. Simon. Psy.D., A.B.P.P. "*Myths of Aging.*" Psychology Today. 2011. https://www.psychologytoday.com/blog/wise/201101/myths-aging

Thank Your Body. "*The ugly truth about vegetable oils (and why they should be avoided).*" Thank Your Body. 2016. http://www.thankyourbody.com/vegetable-oils/

The Defined Dish. "*Bowl of Doom.*" The Defined Dish. 2016. http://www.thedefineddish.com/bowl-of-doom/

Wallance, Michael. M.D. "*The Digestive System & How it Works.*" National Institute of Diabetes and Digestive and Kidney Diseases. 2013. https://www.niddk.nih.gov/health-information/digestive-diseases/digestive-system-how-it-works

Webb, Kelley, Juile. "*Acid Vs. Alkaline in the Body*." Live Strong. 2015. http://www.livestrong.com/article/47620-acid-vs.-alkaline-body/

Wikipedia. "*Myokine*." Wikipedia. 2013. https://en.wikipedia.org/wiki/Myokine

Endnotes

[i] Daily. Science. *"Toba Catastrophe Theory."*
Science Daily.
https://www.sciencedaily.com/terms/toba_catastrophe_theory.htm

[ii] Daily. Science. *"Toba Catastrophe Theory."*
Science Daily.
https://www.sciencedaily.com/terms/toba_catastrophe_theory.htm

[iii] Hötting K., Röder B. *"Beneficial effects of physical exercise on neuroplasticity and cognition."* US National Library of Medicine National Institutes of Health. 2013.
https://www.ncbi.nlm.nih.gov/pubmed/23623982

[iv] R.E. Van Pelt, F. A. Dinneno, D. R. Seals, and P.P. Jones. *"Age-related decline in RMR in physically active men: relation to exercise volume and energy intake."* Am J Physiol Endocrinol Metab, September 2001: 281(3): E633-39.
PubMed PMID:11500320

[v] Tan. Simon. Psy.D., A.B.P.P. *"Myths of Aging."* Psychology Today. 2011.
https://www.psychologytoday.com/blog/wise/201101/myths-aging

[vi] Med-Health. "*Benefits of Muscular Strength.*" Med-Health. 2017. http://www.med-health.net/Benefits-Of-Muscular-Strength.html

[vii] A. R. Brooks-Wilson. „*Genetics of healthy aging and longevity*". Human Genetics. 2013. 132 Issue 12, pp. 1323-38

[viii] Esmonde-White. Miranda. "*Aging Backwards.*"Harper Wave. 2014. pg.15

[ix] Picture I. Surekha. „*Human Cell – Properties, Diagram, Parts, Pictures, Structure.*" Diseases Pictures. 2016. http://diseasespictures.com/human-cell-functions-diagram-parts-pictures-structure/

[x] Surekha. „*Human Cell – Properties, Diagram, Parts, Pictures, Structure.*" Diseases Pictures. 2016. http://diseasespictures.com/human-cell-functions-diagram-parts-pictures-structure/

[xi] Academy. Khan. "*Cellular Respiration.*" Khan Academy. https://www.khanacademy.org/science/biology/cellular-respiration-and-fermentation

[xii] Chan. James. "*Strength Training For Fat Loss: Building A Bigger Engine!*" Body Building. 2016. https://www.bodybuilding.com/content/strength-training-for-fat-loss-building-a-bigger-engine.html

[xiii] Esmonde-White. Miranda. "*Aging Backwards.*"Harper Wave. 2014. pg. 30

[xiv] Campellone. Joseph V. "*Muscle Atrophy.*" Mediline Plus. 2016.

https://medlineplus.gov/ency/article/003188.htm

[xv] Wikipedia. "*Myokine*." Wikipedia. 2013.
https://en.wikipedia.org/wiki/Myokine

[xvi] Wallance, Michael. M.D. "*The Digestive System & How it Works*." National Institute of Diabetes and Digestive and Kidney Diseases. 2013.
https://www.niddk.nih.gov/health-information/digestive-diseases/digestive-system-how-it-works

[xvii] Picture 2. Wallance, Michael. M.D. "*The Digestive System & How it Works*." National Institute of Diabetes and Digestive and Kidney Diseases. 2013.
https://www.niddk.nih.gov/health-information/digestive-diseases/digestive-system-how-it-works

[xviii] Esmonde-White. Miranda. "*Aging Backwards*."Harper Wave. 2014. pg xyz

[xix] Esmonde-White. Miranda. "*Aging Backwards*."Harper Wave. 2014. pg. 130

[xx] Drew. Janice E. "*Cellular Defense System Gene Expression Profiling of Human Whole Blood: Opportunities to Predict Health Benefits in Response to Diet*." Advances in Nutrition. 2012.
http://advances.nutrition.org/content/3/4/499.full

[xxi] Alleva R, Di Donato F, Strafella E, Staffolani S, Nocchi L, Borghi B, Pignotti E, Santarelli L, Tomasetti M. "*Effect of ascorbic acid-rich diet on*

in vivo-induced oxidative stress." Br J Nutr. 2011;Sep 16:1–10.

xxii Crane P. et al. *"Glucose Levels and Risk of Dementia."* NEJM. Sept 2013. Vol 369. National Hospital Discharge Survey (NHDS), National Center for Health Statistics.

xxiii Gangemi, Stephen. *"Elevate Your Cholesterol Profile, Elevate Your Health."* Dr. Gangemi. 2018. http://www.drgangemi.com/health-articles/diet-nutrition/elevate-cholesterol-elevate-health/

xxiv Light. Cooking. *"10 Nutrition Myths."* Cooking Light. 2016. http://www.cookinglight.com/eating-smart/nutrition-101/nutrition-myths-facts/eggs-cholesterol-levels

xxv Webb, Kelley, Juile. *"Acid Vs. Alkaline in the Body."* Live Strong. 2015. http://www.livestrong.com/article/47620-acid-vs.-alkaline-body/

xxvi Dr. Mercola. *"To Protect Your Heart, Your Sodium to Potassium Ratio Is More Important Than Your Overall Salt Intake."* Mercola. 2014. http://articles.mercola.com/sites/articles/archive/2014/08/25/sodium-potassium-ratio.aspx

xxvii S. M. Jeyakumar, A. Vajreswari, B. Sesikeran, and N. V. Giridharan, *"Vitamin A Supplementation Induces Adipose Tissue Loss through Apoptosis in Lean but Not in Obese Rats of the WNIN/OB Strain."* Journal of Molecular Endocrinology. 2005.

http://jme.endocrinology-journals.org/content/35/2/391.full

xxviii Schaefer, Anna. *"Red Wine and Type 2 Diabetes: Is There a Link?"* Health Line. 2017. https://www.healthline.com/health/diabetes/red-wine-and-type-2-diabetes#1

xxix Dr. Axe. *"Is Sugar Bad for You? Here's How It Destroys Your Body."* Dr. Axe – Food is Medicine. 2018. https://draxe.com/is-sugar-bad-for-you/

xxx Gunnars, Kris. *"Is Dairy Bad Or Good?"* Authority Nutrition. 2017. https://authoritynutrition.com/is-dairy-bad-or-good/

xxxi Thank Your Body. *"The ugly truth about vegetable oils (and why they should be avoided)."* Thank Your Body. 2016. http://www.thankyourbody.com/vegetable-oils/

xxxii Mann, Denise. *"Trans Fats: The Science and the Risks."* WebMD. 2018. https://www.webmd.com/diet/features/trans-fats-science-and-risks#1

xxxiii Strawbridge, Holly. *"Artificial sweeteners: sugar-free, but at what cost*?" Harvard Health Publications. 2012. http://www.health.harvard.edu/blog/artificial-sweeteners-sugar-free-but-at-what-cost-201207165030

xxxiv Diven, Alison. *"Cuban Picadillo Lettuce wraps."* The Nourishing Gourmet. 2014. http://www.thenourishinggourmet.com/2014/

07/cuban-picadillo-lettuce-wraps-gf-df-paleo-friendly.html

xxxv Lexi. *"Cajun Garlic Shrimp Noodle Bowls."* Lexi's Clean Kitchen. 2014. http://lexiscleankitchen.com/2014/09/08/cajun-garlic-shrimp-noodle-bowls/

xxxvi The Defined Dish. *"Bowl of Doom."* The Defined Dish. 2016. http://www.thedefineddish.com/bowl-of-doom/

xxxvii Hummusapien. *"The Best Vegan Broccoli Salad."* Hummusapien. 2016. https://www.hummusapien.com/vegan-broccoli-salad/

xxxviii Lexi. *"Italian Style Spaghetti Squash Bake."* Lexi's Clean Kitchen. 2013. http://lexiscleankitchen.com/2013/05/25/italian-style-spaghetti-squash-bake/